Finding Balance

Finding Balance

Healing From a Decade of
Vestibular Disorders

Sue Hickey

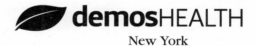

New York

ISBN: 9781936303144
eISBN: 9781617050372
Acquisitions Editor: Noreen Henson
Cover Design: Steven Pisano
Compositor: Absolute Service, Inc.
Printer: Hamilton Printing

Visit our website at www.demoshealth.com

Medical information provided by Demos Health and the author, in the absence of a visit with a healthcare professional, must be considered as an educational service only. This book is not designed to replace a physician's independent judgment about the appropriateness or risks of a procedure or therapy for a given patient. Our purpose is to provide you with information that will help you make your own healthcare decisions.

The information and opinions provided here are believed to be accurate and sound, based on the best judgment available to the authors, editors, and publisher, but readers who fail to consult appropriate health authorities assume the risk of any injuries. The publisher and the author are not responsible for errors or omissions. The publisher and author specifically disclaim all responsibility for any liability, loss, or risk, personal or otherwise, which is incurred as a consequence, directly or indirectly, of the use and application of any of the contents of this book. The editors and publisher welcome any reader to report to the publisher any discrepancies or inaccuracies noticed.

The author does not intend for this information to serve as a substitute for medical advice; any health concerns should be under supervision of a doctor.

Library of Congress Cataloging-in-Publication Data

CIP data is available at the Library of Congress.

Special discounts on bulk quantities of Demos Health books are available to corporations, professional associations, pharmaceutical companies, health care organizations, and other qualifying groups. For details, please contact:

Special Sales Department
Demos Medical Publishing
11 W. 42nd Street
New York, NY 10036
Phone: 800-532-8663 or 212-683-0072
Fax: 212-941-7842
E-mail: rsantana@demosmedpub.com

Made in the United States of America
11 12 13   14   5 4 3 2 1

Contents

Foreword

"If you *listen* carefully to the patient they will tell you the diagnosis."
—*William Osler*

Sue Hickey is an extraordinary person by every measure. Students of vestibular disorders should study her chronicle of complex, multiple, inner ear vestibular disorders. Ms. Hickey has developed a systematic approach to manage vestibular disorders based upon seven distinct stages of her diagnosis, management and outcomes. While individual patient's problems will vary in detail, her practical, systematic and logical approaches will likely help both patient and physician identify and manage one of the most difficult problems in medicine: vestibular disorders.

Among the many problems facing the vestibular patient and their physicians are: 1) no common language exists for reporting perceptions (symptoms) arising from vestibular disturbances, 2) information from the vestibular system is distributed rapidly and subconsciously to all body muscles; the primary distributions are to the eye muscles and to the muscles controlling body center-of-mass in the pelvis. Consequently the patient is limited to attempts to describe the effect(s) of abnormal commands to eye globe (experienced as visual disturbances) and body muscles (usually perceived as imbalance) arising from abnormal vestibular function.

Both patients and physicians are additionally hampered by an inadequate medical education system: vestibular disorders are minimally taught, if taught at all, in medical schools and even residencies. Coupled with a paucity of trained personnel is the limited availability of essential laboratory test facilities. When combined with the tendency to mis-diagnose vestibular disorders as primarily neurological or psychological disorders, the average vestibular patient is in deep trouble. A common example: attributing vestibular symptoms in head trauma patients to brain injury.

Ms. Hickey's book puts forth many important issues and problems that may or may not apply to each individual vestibular patient. However, she points out several principles that affect many patients:

1. There is an important difference between perception and performance from a patient's viewpoint. Specifically, Ms. Hickey was accurate with respect to her perceptions, but tended to futilely 'push through' in attempts to perform, often at great cost in ability to perform activities of daily living consistently.

2. Because of the need to severely restrict physical activity in order to heal perilymph fistulas, neuromuscular de-conditioning results. Ms. Hickey describes some strategies that should help patients deal with both the physical and psychological consequences (especially depression) of restricted physical activity.

3. One of the common medical dictums that must be overcome for patients with multiple vestibular disorders is that the patient's symptoms can be attributed to a single abnormality (a single cause for the abnormal vestibular physiology or pathology). Ms. Hickey had objectively confirmed perilymph fistulas (PLFs), endolymphatic hydrops (ELH) and benign paroxysmal positional nystagmus and vertigo (BPPN & V), all arising at different times and all interacting at some epochs during her clinical course. Consequently, the patient and the physician must attack a series of 'moving targets'. The goal is to determine the major cause of symptoms and attack the most prominent problem first. This task obviously is not simple. For example, PLF patients (especially if undiagnosed for long periods) can develop ELH as a complication. Patients with persistent ELH (including Ménière's disease) develop BPPN. Ms. Hickey's careful logging of symptoms were very helpful in the process of sorting out which conditions were the major source of her symptoms.

Ms. Hickey's book is a well-written treatise of her difficult journey through her suffering and how she dealt with her plight. Her keen observations, approach to identification of her problem(s) and strategies will interest the estimated 69 million patients in the United States with vestibular disorders.[1] More importantly, she presents some techniques and strategies that will help many, if not most, patients cope with vestibular disorders.

Dr. F. Owen Black

---

[1]Agrawal, Y. (2009). Disorders of balance and vestibular function in US adults; Data from the National Health and Nutrition Examination Survey, 2001–2004. *Archives of Internal Medicine, 169*(10), 938–944.

Acknowledgments

My husband, Shelly, was instrumental in helping me learn to accept a new life with vestibular disorders. He was also a primary force supporting my writing and publishing this book, even lending his own insightful thoughts to the narrative. Without his support and assistance this book would not exist.

I am also indebted to Dr. F. Owen Black who provided over a decade of medical treatment for my vestibular disorders. He also volunteered his time to review several versions of the book to assure the medical aspects were correct and helpful to as wide a range of patients as possible. Dr. Bradley Coffey provided especially helpful review of the medical aspects of the book from his perspective of visual rehabilitation. My friend and chiropractor, Paul Hagen, also contributed his valuable perspective.

My vestibular friends—Suzanne, Nancy and Gillie—were especially helpful. Their review of the book confirmed that my story was also their story. Suzanne went even further and assisted me throughout the publication process.

Thank you to Ben who helped research and define the universe of patients, physicians and others in the vestibular community.

To everyone else who read early drafts and provided their feedback, I am very grateful. Without this confirmation that I had a valuable story to tell, I might have put my drafts in a box and filed them away.

Introduction

THE BRAVE NEW WORLD OF VESTIBULAR REALITIES

In December 1997 I was diagnosed with vestibular problems, more commonly known as balance problems. You've probably never heard of vestibular problems; until I had one, neither had I. There are more than ten million people in the United States with debilitating balance problems who may not be aware they have a vestibular disorder, because it is a stealth illness.

By *stealth illness* I mean that vestibular disorders are not widely known; they are not covered in the popular press. There are no medications you might have seen advertised on TV. It's difficult to know you have a vestibular disorder. Vestibular problems also are difficult for a doctor to diagnose, especially when more than one is present. They also are very difficult to fix.

I discovered vestibular disorders the hard way: I flew on an airplane with a cold and woke up the next day dizzy and unable to stand or walk normally. Unbeknownst to me, my ears had been weak my entire life, and the cold had blocked my Eustachian tubes. As a result, I'd sustained tears, called *perilymph fistulas*, in microscopic membranes in my inner ears. During a flight, the eustachian tubes absorb the pressure from altitude changes. When the tubes are blocked because of a cold, the pressure is released through the next available place. Perilymph fistulas can result from these pressure releases. This sounds simple enough, but diagnosing a fistula in the inner ear is akin to trying to fix your car's engine without opening the hood. The rips are microscopic and don't show up on a magnetic resonance imaging or CT scan.

My first symptom, dizziness, is one of the most common medical complaints. It's an indicator of a wide variety of medical conditions, from heart problems to low blood sugar—so common that it's often not helpful in making a diagnosis.

Perhaps it would be more accurate to say that dizziness is not helpful in making a *correct* diagnosis. My diagnosis involved seven doctors, five different medical specialties, and almost two years.

Even when I got to the right doctor—an oto-neurologist specializing in balance problems—a precise diagnosis was not immediate. Many different problems can occur in the inner ear, and those problems have very similar symptoms—dizziness, nausea, headaches, and possibly vertigo. To really complicate matters, several problems often occur at the same time. There is no way to look into the ear and see what is wrong, so diagnosis involves a battery of tests and a sophisticated interpretation of the results. In treating vestibular problems it is important to start with the root cause, the most essential problem, and then work to resolve the next problem, then the next problem, and then the next.

My doctor referred to this process as "peeling the layers" and that's a good description, with one exception: Sometimes the layers don't stay peeled. Vestibular problems can recur; they don't stay resolved, and there you are again, peeling away again. Eventually, I learned to be a better observer of what triggered my symptoms and became an expert on different types of dizziness. Just as an Eskimo needs many words for snow so too does a vestibular patient need a variety of words for dizziness, words and phrases like *tilting, rolling, vibrating, slipping, lightheaded, blurry*, or "movements inside my head."

Nothing in my life prepared me for this illness, let alone an illness that took two years to diagnose. My life was transformed by my journey through the healing process. A multitude of small (and some not-so-small!) setbacks compounded the challenges. It wasn't all bleak, though: Serendipitous events and connections materialized regularly to counterbalance the setbacks.

The healing process required all of my hard-earned life skills and forced me to develop even more of those skills. One of the most helpful things I relied on to foster healing was writing in my journal. For more than thirty years, I'd counted on my journal to help me through difficult emotional times. When I got sick, I regularly chronicled what was happening and my thoughts and feelings as a way to chart my progress. My journal entries represented a way to express myself, unencumbered by the need to be socially acceptable or to avoid upsetting someone. By writing down whatever came into my head, I was generally able to see problems more clearly and gain some needed perspective. I was also able to look back over the weeks and months of writing and determine whether I was making any progress. When I was unable to recall how I was feeling at any given moment, the journal provided an eyewitness account. I rely on my journal to tell the story of my healing process.

In telling this story I also rely on the notes I kept about every interaction with a medical practitioner. (This was a useful practice from my corporate life—keeping notes about meetings for future reference.) I kept extensive records on my symptoms, as best I understood them. The record keeping became very valuable after my diagnosis, when I was better educated about what symptoms to record.

A few years into the healing process, my notes and journal revealed several distinct stages. Early in my recovery, there was *denial*, and then *confusion and frustration*. After I was diagnosed, I relaxed into *surrender* and later emerged into *experimenting* and then *adapting*. Once I began *managing* my recovery, it was not long before I reached the final stage of healing: *acceptance*. As with most stages in life, there was considerable overlap, no helpful bold demarcations. Also, I saw the stages in hindsight, when I had some perspective and distance. At the time, events or turning points helped me recognize a new phase, but I seemed to understand their full importance only in hindsight. Also, of course, about the time I truly began to understand each phase I moved on to the next one and was grappling with the new lessons there.

Finding Balance is the story of my journey through healing: the medical facts as well as my personal perspectives. It is a story of physical changes that transformed me not just physically but emotionally and spiritually. It is a story of loss but also of gain. In its simplest form, it is the story of my recovery from the cold and the airplane flight in 1996. But it's really about nothing less than restoring balance to my life.

Finding Balance

1

Losing Balance

MARCH 1996–APRIL 1996

Revolutionary change can enter our lives disguised as inconsequential events. In March 1996 I got a cold, a cold like the dozens of colds I'd weathered throughout my life, infinitely forgettable. This cold appeared the day before a hastily scheduled trip to North Carolina. Unlike the cold, my reason for the trip was memorable: I was going for a short visit with my father before spending a few days touring possible nursing home facilities for him.

I arrived in Raleigh, North Carolina, to a large, frigid hotel room. It was after midnight local time but only 9:00 p.m. Portland, Oregon, time. I needed to get up early for the three-hour drive to the mountains to reach my father, so I took an aspirin to ease the headache and settled in with a very dull book. The trip from west to east has always been difficult for me, and this one was as well—too early for sleep and of course too many thoughts about the reason I was here.

My father was slowly succumbing to Alzheimer's disease. When I finally drove down the single-track road to his little house on the mountain-top, I saw him in the front yard, pitching golf balls into a net. He was confused by the strange car, but then there was his huge grin the moment he recognized me. I cherished every minute of the next ten hours. Dad was completely lucid and full of his usual jokes and stories. We walked around the hills and then simply sat and talked for hours. These moments alone together had been few and far between in recent years.

March 17, 1996

It was a wonderful, reassuring visit. He immediately wanted to sit down and talk about Alzheimer's: What did I know about it? Was it really bad to drink if you had Alzheimer's? How did you get it? He described what it felt like to him . . . frustrating. He said it was not that he didn't know who I was but sometimes he could not recall the word for my name. That happens also when he is talking in general, he has to stop because he can't find the words. He is aware of having good days and bad days—or being restless at night . . . It was odd but it seemed he cared more and was more interested in my life, my sister's lives, than ever. He admitted he sometimes "practiced" for my visits and that he often fakes it or remains quiet if he loses the thread. But he wasn't losing any threads at that point.

He said he did not think it was getting much worse. I see him working very hard to make that so. Even though the decline is undeniable—he is still himself. His personality—that impish, feisty character—is very much there. I'm so pleased to see him fight so hard.

As Dad got more and more tired, he became less and less lucid. By the time I left he was completely focused on his nighttime routine and barely noticed my leaving. As my stepmother helped him into his pajamas, he appeared not to recognize me. Seeing that change, just over the course of the ten hours I was there, it seemed clear the move to a nursing home was not *if,* but *when.*

That evening, after my sister Anne finished work, she drove up and rendezvoused with me at the local Holiday Inn. She arrived with information on the care facilities in the surrounding area. We wanted to visit four or five different places to get a feel for where Dad would be most comfortable. We were both professional women: strong, analytical, and pragmatic. We had checklists and a businesslike approach. No matter how professional or strong we were, though, this was unfamiliar territory, filled with substantial emotional challenges.

The next day, we repeated the details of Dad's condition at each new facility, toured the Alzheimer's unit, and imagined giving him up to each place. We were relieved to find two wonderful places: one with a long waiting list, the other with one immediate opening. Our stepmother and other two sisters would be involved in any decision, so we asked questions, noted our impressions, and kept hoping this move wouldn't be necessary: Dad was clearly functioning better than the other residents we saw.

After completing our visits, we drove back to Raleigh, where Anne lived and where I'd catch my flight home. We were encouraged about the possibilities and worn out from all the emotion. My head was stuffy and aching, and my eyes were red and swollen. I could no longer distinguish my cold sniffles from the effects of having been repeatedly moved to tears. I didn't even think about my cold on the flight to Portland as I tried to shift gears away from the heart-wrenching focus of North Carolina. My husband, Shelly, was away on business, so I was coming home to an empty house—except for my cat, Looey, and my dog, Bunkee—and a very busy week. I was exhausted when I arrived at home and realized that my cold had gotten worse. As I climbed into bed, I trusted that a good night's sleep would work wonders, as always.

Not this time.

I woke up groggy and still exhausted. When I tried to get up, the room spun wildly. I sat back on the bed to avoid a fall and waited for the room to stop moving. After resting a few minutes and catching my breath, I tried getting up and walking slowly. After a few halting steps, I realized that if I walked slowly, concentrating with every step, I could tolerate the spinning. I showered and took a very brief walk with Bunkee. I thought I felt a little better; the world was moving a bit less erratically.

I was the chief operating officer of the Bonneville Power Administration, a multistate electric utility company. It was a challenging job even in quiet times, but now the utility—in fact, the entire electric utility industry—was in crisis because of impending deregulation. Every utility was working overtime to lower costs, reduce staff, and reorient the business toward the more market-based approach that deregulation would bring. My job was to lead the effort to reduce staff and spending in a careful, strategic way. Every day there was another urgent task or critical decision that could not be delayed.

I thought about staying home from work the next morning, but I was scheduled to lead an employee meeting and present a business strategy to a group of financial rating agencies for an upcoming bond sale. My absence would mean canceling the employee meeting on very short notice, and there were several important things I needed to say there. The rating agency visit was similarly critical, and no substitutes were readily available. I wasn't bleeding, I wasn't throwing up, and no bones were broken. Calling in sick seemed like an overreaction to something that would surely clear up soon. I decided to press forward with my busy day at work.

As I got into the car, I realized I was dizzy every time I moved my eyes, not just my head. I had to drive to get to work, so I took local streets instead of the 405 freeway and tried not to turn my head very rapidly or very often. As I walked in slowly from the parking lot, I remembered similar symptoms a year earlier—dizziness, a slight spinning sensation, and nausea. I'd gone to the doctor, and he concluded it was a virus. He assured me it would clear up in a few weeks. It had.

I had no reason to think this dizziness wouldn't follow the same pattern I'd experienced the year before: a mild inconvenience not significant enough to disrupt the demands of my normal life. For the next few days I still felt dizzy and totally exhausted, but I was convinced that it would all soon clear up. I pushed the dizziness into the background, walked around slowly and "gutted it out."

Pushing other parts of my life into the background to accommodate the requirements of my career was a well-established personal pattern. Despite lifelong attempts to balance my work and personal life, I was continuously attracted to demanding jobs and work situations.

Because Shelly was not home at the time, I could get away with this self-destructive behavior more readily. By the end of the week Shelly was home, and it didn't take him long at all to see I was in a tailspin.

April 2, 1996

Sunday Shelly called my bluff. He challenged my driven behavior and it all fell apart—my deep sense of sadness and sorrow about Dad and my avoidance of that sadness by burying myself in work. The next day the dizziness was even worse accompanied by loud ear ringing and nausea.

I got worse over the weekend. I was dizzy and constantly nauseated. The room spun for longer periods. My ears rang loudly, and it seemed like I wasn't hearing well with my right ear. On Monday I made an appointment with the same doctor who had treated me so successfully the year before.

Shelly escorted me to the doctor's office because I was feeling very, very tired and the dizziness made it hard to walk. We sat in the waiting room, and I felt completely flat, emotionless. I didn't even have the energy to think. Looking back, I realize I was also completely trusting. I believed the doctor would, of course, know what was wrong and give me a prescription for medication to fix it. The complete cure might take a few weeks, but it was unlikely I would even remember this slight inconvenience six months from now. Every medical experience in my life up to this point reinforced that expectation.

In the examining room I described my symptoms to the doctor: a cold-type flu turning into a week-long bout with dizziness, some spinning, constant nausea, a deafening ringing in my right ear, and total absence of energy. I also mentioned that I had not been hearing well out of my right ear. The doctor was supportive and understanding, as always. Everything went according to the familiar pattern until he administered the routine hearing test. I couldn't hear out of my right ear at all! I could see that the doctor viewed this development with increased concern, but I was in a fog of fatigue and dizziness.

My doctor's office is in a large local hospital with a full range of services available on a moment's notice. He wanted to rule out the worst possibility— that the hearing loss was caused by a tumor—as quickly as possible. He ordered a magnetic resonance imaging scan (MRI) immediately, and within fifteen minutes I was out of his office, down two long flights of stairs and wandering through seemingly endless dull green, empty corridors until I reached the MRI room. I was inside the long cold MRI tube before I could get nervous. I glanced at Shelly through the glass. He looked nervous.

Shelly: When Sue came out to the waiting room to tell me she had to go "right now" to get an MRI to check for a brain tumor, my heart started racing. I remember taking both of her hands and asking "What did he say?" As she explained his thinking in a little more detail I caught my breath. I remember saying something like "Good thinking. Let's go eliminate that as an option immediately." Maybe that calmed us both down a little, or at least offered us both a façade we could slip behind.

The walk down to the MRI room was difficult. We were winding through the below-ground floors of a hospital complex that clearly had a series of buildings added over time, attached to the old hospital, with lefts and rights and short steps down and up. It took forever. We had to keep ourselves from breaking into a trot. Sometimes, at the T-junctions, the signs were a little off to the side, and we had to walk left to see the sign, and then backtrack and walk right to get going again in the right direction. There was no one else in the corridor. We ran into no one.

Then we found the MRI room. Sue handed them the doctor's request form and filled out two others for them. She barely had time to turn around from the reception window, sit down, and adjust her coat before they called her in, I kissed her cheek and told her not to worry, and she disappeared through the door.

The magazine pile consisted only of *Ladies' Home Journals* and decorating and children's magazines. I asked the receptionist how long it would take. She said 45 minutes if they got her in right away.

Why did they take her then if they weren't going to start immediately, I wondered?

I flipped through a magazine, not even looking at the pages, staring at the floor in front of me, trying to think of any friends I knew who were doctors, who I could ask what they thought of this, trying to breath deeply and slow down my heartbeat, trying to think positive thoughts, trying to climb up from the abyss.

The MRI was a turning point: not because the results were positive; they weren't, and not because it led to a diagnosis; it didn't. The MRI was a turning point because it was the start of a new medical experience. It was the first of many tests and procedures done to rule out specific conditions. "Process of elimination" was the primary diagnostic strategy. We weren't figuring out what I had, we were figuring out what I didn't have. Unlike the childhood game of Twenty Questions, there was little logic to the process. It probably would have helped if I could have seen that fact and all its resultant frustrations at an early stage.

The next week my doctor referred me to an ear, nose, and throat specialist who confirmed my hearing loss and balance problems after administering a battery of tests. The hearing tests were sophisticated measurements conducted in soundproof booths. By contrast, the balance tests were rudimentary maneuvers like walking in a straight line or standing and lifting one leg. It didn't matter—I couldn't pass even the simplest of them. When the specialist spoke to me after these tests, he focused only on my hearing loss and whether it would recover. I was speechless. He paid no attention to my balance problems. He offered no explanation for the cause of the hearing loss. He did not provide any advice on how I might improve my overall condition. He did not even address the fatigue, the nausea, or the lack of balance. He offered no advice about further tests or medical expertise I should pursue. I was furious! Even with my overwhelming fatigue and fear, I could feel how angry I was. I remained angry with this physician for years. He became the focus of my disappointment and growing sense of abandonment by the medical community.

April 22, 1996

I am nauseous all the time, exhausted at any activity and real weepy and emotional. I get dizzy when I bend down or recline, can't hear out of my right ear—and I guess just flat depressed to feel so bad for so long—4 to 6 weeks. I am really struggling.

At the same time as I want to get back to a normal work schedule—a signal of normalcy and strength—I am dreading it on an

*emotional level. I just don't feel very strong, very resilient, very patient.
I am really struggling with my health and with how my work and the
balance of my life play into that. . . . No clarity here, mostly sadness.*

I had no idea what was wrong, let alone how to fix it, and apparently
no one else did, either. I was still counting on this dizziness to clear up like
it had a few years ago, but it had now lasted six weeks, and there were no
signs of improvement. I hoped I could just endure the symptoms and wait
for whatever was wrong to go away or get better.

Not knowing what else to do, I continued to do what I always did:
I kept on going. I was not able to work my usual sixty to sixty-five hours a
week, but I tried. I tried to keep up the usual social engagements. I dragged
myself out to walk the dog several times a day. Shelly frequently traveled for
business, and when he was not home I collapsed in the evening—getting
into bed at 6:30 or 7:00 p.m. Work, sleep, walk the dog, and wonder: "What
is wrong with me?"

Speaking From Experience: Tips to Make Your Journey Easier

1. Although life was largely a blur after the airplane trip, I kept recording
   the same symptoms—dizziness, spinning, nausea, deafness, and fatigue.
   These symptoms were the only clues I had to solve the mystery of what
   was wrong. Tracking symptoms—regardless of whether you understand
   them—is an essential first step in getting a diagnosis. List as much
   information as you can about the symptom: the severity (using a range
   of 1–10); what you were doing that might have caused the symptom;
   how long it lasted; and what, if anything, relieves the symptom.

2. Until my internist and the ear, nose, and throat specialist were
   unable to provide a diagnosis, I never imagined such a possibility. In
   my experience as a patient, I was a passive reporter and the doctor
   provided the knowledge, insight, and direction—the answer. It took
   me years, and an illness that is confounding to diagnose, to break
   myself of this old habit and become an active participant in my health
   care. Before a definitive diagnosis is made, it's hard to feel part of a
   team. However, clarity about your symptoms as well as an organized
   and focused effort to find the right doctor is critical. The Vestibular
   Disorders Association (www.vestibular.org) has a Web site with general
   information resources as well as a list of medical practitioners in each
   state. It's a good place to start the search.

2

Denial: Is Anything Really Wrong With Me?

APRIL 1996–AUGUST 1996

Throughout that first month of my symptoms, I worked very hard to present the appearance of normalcy. Being a very private person, I simply did not want to reveal my troubles and concerns to others. Without a diagnosis or any plausible theory about what was wrong, the question "What's wrong with you" could be answered only with "I don't know." Without a diagnosis I didn't know if I was really sick—at least, that's how it felt to me. That feeling grew over the months.

One night I went to the symphony with one of my oldest friends, my college boyfriend, Paul, who had become a chiropractor. We were walking to my car after the concert in the dark, in the drizzle that is common to Portland in the spring. He asked how I was feeling. I said I felt like someone who'd lived through a stroke. In addition to the general dizziness and fatigue, the right side of my body felt like it was sagging. I struggled to walk. I immediately regretted being so forthcoming because it seemed so overly dramatic, so clearly a cry for sympathy.

Paul urged me to aggressively pursue a diagnosis and treatment. He emphasized that conditions that are not addressed either become chronic or appear to abate only to reemerge in much more serious, life-threatening forms later. The word *life-threatening* didn't really register through the omnipresent fog and fatigue, but his prompting and concern were what I needed to hear.

I was 48 at the time and had always been physically vigorous and active. I had been a vegetarian for 25 years. I ran, hiked, skied, and sailed. I liked being active, and I wanted to stay active my whole life. Paul gave me the wake-up call I needed. It was the same wake up Shelly had been shouting but for some reason I had refused to hear. I recognized that I had to start listening to the people who cared about me. They saw my condition more objectively than I did.

My first step was to see the naturopath Paul recommended. Naturopaths prefer to use natural remedies, such as herbs and foods, rather than surgery or synthetic drugs. The naturopath immediately diagnosed a systemic infection and prescribed a series of homeopathic remedies. I saw him every two weeks for the next nine months. At each appointment we discussed my response to the remedy I was trying and he used a fascinating piece of equipment that electronically measured responses at the standard acupuncture pressure points to identify the current state of my health.

The naturopath referred to my condition as "a chronic fatigue–related syndrome." This was the first time I had heard the term *chronic fatigue* spoken by a medical professional. Until then, all I knew about chronic fatigue was what I read in the paper or saw on TV. These accounts characterized the condition as something that happened to driven, Type A personality people for unexplainable reasons. These reports insinuated that the condition was psychosomatic. I didn't much like the Type A label, or the psychosomatic implications, but it was a relief to have at least some sense of what might be wrong.

As the weeks wore on and the physical fatigue, constant nausea, and dizziness did not abate, I got very depressed. On top of the other symptoms, the emotional drain of depression was unwelcome, to say the least. So far my list of symptoms seemed to just get longer. The prospect of adding depression was . . . depressing! The naturopath introduced me to homeopathic St. John's Wort. He had been having me try a different homeopathic remedy every other week. I wanted to believe it was helping—that we were on the trail of an elusive illness—but I didn't notice any positive effects.

St. John's Wort was the first remedy I noticed that had any effect at all on any of my symptoms. From May 1996 on, through the worst times of my illness, I relied on St. John's Wort to push the depression into the background. This remedy was essential to my healing because it removed the hopelessness and lack of motivation.

*　　*　　*

I continued to work as many hours as I could through March and April of 1996. National developments in electricity deregulation were overtaking the Bonneville Power Administration reorganization I'd worked so hard on in 1994. It was now necessary to completely separate the transmission and generation functions in the organization. These changes were not as traumatic as the previous ones had been; employees were used to the idea of change, and the realignments were more modest. The good news was that when generation and transmission functions were in separate organizations, even if all still under the Bonneville Power Administration roof, the organization was more efficient and responsibilities were clearer. To create those separate organizations, many of the executives needed to be reassigned to new positions. This meant more tension for the colleagues with whom I worked most closely. It was also my responsibility to make the decisions regarding the organization and the placement of executives.

In general, leadership responsibilities were quite evenly shared within the group of executives. Each executive led his or her own area, and the executives as a group collaborated on the broad decisions and issues affecting the entire organization. This collaboration allowed us to make decisions, communicate, and resolve issues rapidly. My area of responsibility included deciding who would be responsible for what within the organization. This meant all executive reorganization and shifts in responsibility were my area to supervise, a particularly significant leadership challenge!

It was difficult but I continued to work through all these planned changes and shifts in responsibility until my naturopath recommended a trial month away from work and deep rest to assist in my recovery from "chronic fatigue." I had now been struggling for almost two months with these perplexing health issues. As I limped through April, I predicted that the major decisions and actions in the reorganization would occur in June and July. I decided to try a medical leave in May to see if I could shake the symptoms. My boss readily supported the recommendation. He saw how sick I was.

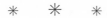

When I actually took the month of medical leave in May, I didn't know what to do with myself. It was a relief to sleep longer and to rest for long periods each day, but sitting around feeling sorry for myself wasn't going to help much, either. I'd never overcome a challenge by just lying on the couch before so I set out to build a healthy, revitalizing plan of action.

I started to meditate regularly again. Over the years, meditation had served as a refuge and source of strength and solace. The stillness involved in meditating cleansed me and gave me strength. It was the deepest rest I knew. Meditation and journal writing had been the strongest medicine to heal whatever had ailed me in the past. Naturally, I turned again to these old friends.

I also knew I'd need to engage in physical activity. Breathing deeply and using my body rather than my mind built up a different source of strength than my usual willpower. In the past, running had been my sweat mechanism of choice, but now running sapped too much energy. I started to walk. I couldn't walk very far or very fast without getting dizzy and tired, so what I did was more like meandering, but my dog Bunkee and I made our rounds, slowly, around the neighborhood several times a day. The walks cleared my head and reduced the nausea.

I'd envisioned gardening as ideal for building strength gently, and after a long winter of gray and rain, and a typically cold and disappointing April, May was a gardener's delight. I was soon disappointed to find how little I could do without getting fatigued. My vision of relaxed gardening met the reality of hard dirty work: It sapped energy rather than providing a restful change. The gardening vision turned into a disappointment and failure.

All through May I found it difficult to stop thinking about things I should be doing because I was not spending all my time working—errands, household chores, reconnecting with friends. I applied my old standards of accomplishment to what should have been a restful activity and I ruined it for myself. Soon I realized that one month would not be sufficient for a full recovery.

The medical leave did not cure the problem, but it helped me see the relationship between my workload and the effects of the sickness. The less I tried to do, the better I felt. Even though I was still tired, still dizzy, and still nauseated when I got up in the morning, and I was still experiencing constant muscle aches and an intermittent sore throat, the intensity seemed less; the magnitude was reduced. The month away from work was my first real sense that work sapped the energy I needed to get well. I now needed to devise strategies for accommodating the illness—to get on with my life in a way that accommodated the fatigue and the dizziness while I still hoped it would go away on its own accord.

During May, while I was working a few hours a week at home, I began to recognize that I needed to loosen my grip on the reins of my life. I began to think about working differently—not more or less, but differently.

My normal work schedule included running most of the ten to twelve meetings I attended every day. In all my interactions with groups of employees, as well as smaller private meetings, I was very conscious of the need to be a good leader, worthy of their trust and respect. This need to be a good leader was a constant pressure; there was no down time, no letup. It was like always being on stage, in character.

In addition, the way I chose to work compounded the energy drain.

May 22, 1996

It seems like I understand what is going on (at work) very well working 15 hours a week at home. This could mean I don't need to be involved in nearly as many meetings and interactions, especially if it is merely to be informed. If I am clear about my objective and purpose in each interaction that could heighten my impact and lessen the interactions.

Things are not hopeless unless I think I am solely responsible for correcting every detail. I need to hang back more and let others take the initiative. I need to wait to see if someone else will raise the point. Watching and waiting takes less energy, others learn more.

I went back to work with a new resolve to work smarter and thus get well faster.

It didn't work. My condition quickly deteriorated right back to where I'd been before the medical leave even though I limited myself to working no more than forty hours per week. Except for the recovery of my hearing, all of my other symptoms persisted.

June 26, 1996

I had some very low days the end of last week and over the weekend. Very tired, very off balance, and nauseated in the morning. It was hard to make it through work: re-engineering decisions, group meetings on next steps and the executive feedback. I got home Thursday and Friday with no energy—even to eat or talk. It is impossible to describe how bad and lifeless those times are.

I am writing all this down because I can't tell if I am getting better or worse since I started back to work. I am working close to 40 hours a week and that is my limit, although some of it is at home reading. Depression appears to be lessening.

Also as a result of the medical leave and the opportunity to reflect and search for next steps, I began to record my symptoms every day. I hoped this would help me identify a pattern.

June 18, 1996

Pretty nauseated in the morning, and dizzy. Made myself walk 1 mile—felt a bit better. Worked 9 to 3. Didn't feel good when got home but walked 2 miles. Then rested. Slept hard. Real physically tired. Muscles sore. Ear ringing.

Throughout these months, even with all the symptoms, I had a hard time thinking of myself as sick. I certainly did not look sick. I had no external signs of physical infirmity: no broken bones, no wheelchair, no radical treatment regimen. I was still quite physically active. I walked twice a day, often for a total of four or five miles. Moving around seemed to make me feel better—more stable, with better equilibrium. (Later I figured out that if I limited my walks to about three miles I felt good; any more made me tired for days.) I was even running periodically from sheer force of habit.

I had always thought of sickness as something acute. It stopped you in your tracks and landed you in bed. Sickness meant constant pain and suffering, extreme treatment approaches, visible disabilities. I had difficulty thinking of myself as sick because my condition did not match any of those expectations. Until my medical leave in May, most people at work were not even aware I was experiencing any difficulty. Soon after I returned to work, people began to approach me and wish me well. Many of these people were sick themselves. To my eyes they struggled with far more serious challenges than I. It was inspirational to hear their stories and very moving that they discussed their vulnerability so openly with me. I felt like a fraud. I was unable to accept that I was sick like they were. Only later did I understand this was one of the clearest indicators I was in the denial stage.

In many ways I was sleepwalking through a series of critical decisions and actions at work. A large amount of informal mediating was needed during this stage in the reorganization, and I was the natural choice for mediator. I was able to focus my energy to make a high-priority decision or engage in a sensitive mediation, but it was adrenaline that was helping me through each crisis. My energy was low and easily depleted. After each emotional session, I collapsed. I literally came home and stared at the wall or, even worse, cried. Shelly was working very hard and traveling all the time—I think he had double platinum frequent-flyer miles on three airlines—but I was glad he was not there to see me break down and cry. I even tried to hide it from the dog and the cat because it invariably made them feel they had done something wrong.

*   *   *

In May, Shelly and I went for a long walk with some friends, Jacob and Tina, who also were the proud owners of a young dog. During the walk through Forest Park, a large wooded park in our neighborhood, we talked about how I was feeling and what I was doing about it. Tina was a nurse, and Jacob was a vascular surgeon. He became visibly agitated as I described my symptoms and the naturopath who was treating me. He was both concerned about my lingering problems and offended that I was not seeing a "real" doctor. He took up the challenge of finding me a "real" doctor and clearly viewed my case as some sort of test of honor for traditional medicine.

This was not the first time I'd seen there was a difference of view, sometimes bordering on mistrust and disrespect, between traditional doctors and alternative practitioners. My first-hand experience was fairly positive with both types of treatment. I certainly did not rule out the possibility that traditional medicine had something to offer, and I appreciated Jacob's willingness to provide a medical referral. Usually I would have counted on my internist for a referral, but I was still angry and disappointed about my internist's referral to the useless ear, nose, and throat doctor.

Within a few days, Jacob referred me to a neurologist he had recently consulted for one of his patients. When I called the office to make an appointment, I felt a bit conspiratorial circumventing the usual health system channels. It also seemed more than a bit odd to be referred to a neurologist by a vascular surgeon. In these early days of seeking a diagnosis I was overly concerned with proper protocol, timid in the face of patients with real problems and doctors with real conditions to treat.

After I recounted my symptoms to the neurologist, starting with the cold virus, he administered a few simple neurological tests. I stretched one arm out in front of me and then, with my eyes closed, brought my finger to my nose. For another test I had to walk a straight line, placing my heel up against the toe of my other foot. I failed every test. I could not do any of these simple things. I was embarrassed and surprised—embarrassed because these actions were so simple and elementary I could not believe I couldn't do them and surprised because these simple tests were one of the first things that externally confirmed how I felt every day.

The neurologist said the tests revealed physical conditions caused by an "inflammation of the eighth cranial nerve." Inflammations of the eighth cranial nerve caused imbalance, hearing fluctuation, and something he referred to as *emotional incontinence.*

The neurologist said the tests revealed physical conditions caused by an "inflammation of the eighth cranial nerve." Inflammations of the eighth cranial nerve caused imbalance, hearing fluctuation, and something he referred to as *emotional incontinence.* Although he was not certain what was causing the inflammation, he was not convinced it was chronic fatigue. He recommended I complete a battery of simple baseline tests to see whether we could find the cause of the inflammation. He recommended testing for lupus and for Lyme disease as well as a chest X-ray and a blood sedimentation rate test. If all of these tests were negative and the debilitating symptoms continued, he recommended a lumbar puncture—a spinal tap—to rule out the possibility that I was in the early stages of multiple sclerosis. He emphasized that he would not want to proceed with the lumbar puncture until all of the other possible causes had been ruled out.

Emotional incontinence is a sterile professional term for what you and I would call unexplained crying jags. At the slightest provocation, I burst into tears. I had never been the type of person who cried readily, and when I did cry I found it uncomfortable and recovered—or covered my feelings—as rapidly as possible. Over the past few months I had been moved to tears continually: a conflict at work, a sad film, a mistake my puppy made, or perhaps nothing at all. Sometimes it was not just a few well-concealed tears and I sobbed on and on for minutes at a time. Of all the symptoms that made me feel out of control, this emotional incontinence was at the head of the list. Several of my close friends had suggested menopause as the culprit, but I had gone through those changes a few years before with no difficulty. Finding out that this was a part of an illness and not a sudden personality change was a huge relief. This relief caused me to realize that somewhere in my fog I was concerned about Alzheimer's disease. Personality changes are part of Alzheimer's disease, and with my family history I was terrified of early-onset Alzheimer's.

In addition to this preliminary diagnosis and the helpful insights on emotional incontinence, the neurologist gave me a tutorial on the state of affairs in the medical bureaucracy. He advised me to become my own advocate and to seek the assistance of my internist. He emphasized that it was my responsibility to determine the direction of my care.

The emphasis the neurologist placed on becoming my own advocate reinforced the messages I was getting from Shelly and my medical friends. The doctor said I would have a difficult time finding an internist who was not influenced by the new gatekeeper role brought on by the HMO system. I headed back to my internist to update him on my progress and pursue the tests the neurologist had recommended. I now understood the approach of ruling out more exotic medical conditions as my primary method of diagnosis.

It may have been my imagination, but I felt my internist was a bit defensive when I reported on my appointment with the neurologist. At the very least he was curious about how I happened to see this particular neurologist. My attempt to explain made me quite uncomfortable. I was still hesitant about taking the leadership role in my own health care. I had always relied totally on the advice of my doctors. For so many years my role was to report symptoms and wait for doctors to solve the problem, or at least suggest the next step. The internist grudgingly ordered the tests indicated by the neurologist. He believed I was suffering from chronic fatigue and expressed his doubt that the tests would reveal anything new.

One by one the results came back: negative. It was hard to see this as the good news it was. I certainly didn't want to have lupus or any of the other things they tested for; I wasn't even sure what some of the potential conditions were. I just wanted to find a specific cause of the inflammation and then of course a remedy, so I could just get well.

In between medical appointments and tests I continued to work, although my heart and mind were not in it.

July 8, 1996

Another pattern I want to note is a feeling of disappointment and lack of satisfaction with my work. This has been the case for the last several months and I can't sort out the sickness from reality. I don't feel strong, I don't feel engaged, and in general I don't feel interested.

I am confused about whether I am simply "sick" and "tired" . . . and should put my observations on hold until I feel physically better . . . or whether the job is a contributing factor to my physical difficulties. It is clear it is not helping. So this confusion is compounding my concern that I am not getting well—that I am struggling through.

Speaking From Experience: Tips to Make Your Journey Easier

1. After a few months, I noticed some additional symptoms. I felt like I was in a fog and had difficulty concentrating. The muscles in my arms and legs ached constantly and I was surprisingly emotional, especially when I was tired. I still couldn't find any rational connection between the symptoms, so all I could do was list them. I got a separate calendar for recording symptoms and dutifully listed them daily. In retrospect, I might have understood some patterns—like the influence of weather or too much exercise—if I'd summarized my symptoms each week.

2. During this early experience I began to identify activities that made me feel worse—too much walking or running and too many hours at work. I also noticed that rest and meditation made me feel better. I didn't do a good job at cutting back, but I began to observe some causes and effects. This was the very beginning of learning to live with limits.

3. Throughout this period I was deeply conflicted about whether I was really sick. This was compounded by my inability to tell whether I was feeling any better—or worse. My daily list of symptoms was getting longer, so that was the evidence I relied on to tell the story. This confusion—combined with the fatigue—kept me from being as aggressive as I needed to be in seeking a diagnosis. The sooner you realize your health is your top priority, the better.

3

The Pendulum Swings Wildly

SEPTEMBER 1996–JANUARY 1997

In late August I suddenly started to see flashing white lights. The episodes came and went several times a day. The worst part was the flashes partially blinded me. The lights blocked out patches of my field of vision in both eyes. It first occurred as an allergic reaction to a medication, but it continued after the medication stopped. Much later, I learned that these flashes are referred to as a *visual migraine*. Visual events like these frequently precede migraines; they are an early warning signal. However, I wasn't experiencing any migraines—yet.

Alarmed by these new developments, and frustrated with the general lack of progress, I scheduled another appointment with the neurologist. Over the summer I had finished all the tests he requested—I completed my goal—and the symptoms had not gone away. I felt hopeless. Was I going to feel like this forever? At the very least, it was time to rule out more serious conditions, such as early-stage multiple sclerosis. The neurologist agreed there was no progress, and we scheduled the spinal tap for early September.

In retrospect, I realize that I was an idiot about this procedure. The neurologist warned me that some people experience severe headaches and are unable to stand up for days after a spinal tap. He described the type of person who encounters difficulty: women who have a slight build. He was telling me I was at risk for a difficult recovery from the test, but I was not paying attention. I still saw myself as a person who sailed through physical challenges—who recovered more quickly, who experienced the least pain, who healed at record speed. Also, I was determined to have this procedure. In my quest for a diagnosis and treatment, it was the next step. After only six months as a sick person I clung tightly to these old perceptions of myself, believing firmly that these last six months were only an aberration.

The spinal tap is a creepy procedure—barbaric, in fact. A needle is literally inserted into the spine to extract spinal fluid for testing. My spinal tap was relatively simple and fast. I felt no pain during the procedure or for hours afterwards. It was especially reassuring when my neurologist called in the evening to ask how I was doing and I was able to truthfully report that I felt fine. I planned to take a few days off of work to recover: The procedure was done on a Thursday, and I expected to be back at work the following Monday.

However, on Friday I was weak and achy. The doctor had told me it would be necessary to lie flat on my back for a few days. This was just a bit misleading. "Flat on your back" did not mean sitting up in bed, reading, it meant totally flat—no pillow, no incline whatsoever, totally flat. Actually, I could lie totally flat on my stomach, too, but that didn't provide a lot of relief or entertainment. Deviating from this meant an instantaneous and severe lightning bolt of pain down my spine. If it is possible to have a migraine along your spinal cord, this was it. It did not go away after a few seconds; it got worse and worse the whole time I remained vertical. At one low moment several days into this pattern, I seriously thought I was dying. I thought it had to be some severe, life-threatening problem that was causing such pain. These fleeting thoughts of death were high drama in my life of flat emotions and mind-numbing dizziness. But they did get the point across—this was unbearable pain, relentless pain.

However, on Tuesday morning I just decided I was ready to go back to work. I had already recuperated one day longer than I expected, and enough was enough. I got up and got in the shower. Within a minute I'd collapsed on the side of the tub. The pain was unbearable; I was shaking and sick to my stomach. I almost passed out. I crawled back to bed and lay there crying for at least an hour. In the midst of this nightmare I experienced a genuine epiphany. I saw my limit. Pushing through, toughing it out, was not helping me anymore.

As I lay flat on my back, I asked myself why I was pushing so hard to get back to work. In a flash of insight, I understood that I was afraid I would miss something. Even after a twenty-five-year career I thought I needed to be at every meeting, read every piece of information, talk to every interested party, in order to be good enough. At almost the same instant, I realized this was ridiculous! It was a rare moment of total clarity. I saw right through to the conclusion: At this point in my career my experience, and the insights my experience provided, were the most valuable things I could contribute. It was no longer my job to read everything, talk to everyone, be the most prepared. I was good enough.

September 25, 1996

Maybe more important, I feel I have really learned a lesson—I saw my limit, I saw how insanely hard I push myself and I gave up. At this point I feel I let go on a deep level—at the level of my lifelong need to push myself and everyone else to make it happen. . . . I hope to hang on to this lesson. It is not necessary or desirable to get back in that place.

This was a huge epiphany. I realized I needed to change. When I heard the results from the spinal tap were normal, the whole process seemed tragic, bordering on comic. I was tired, nauseous, and dizzy, but I was functioning. It was ironic: I had pushed hard for a diagnostic test that made me feel far worse than the illness, whatever it was. The real comic gesture was to come next.

In early October I called to schedule a follow-up appointment with my neurologist and learned he was on extended medical leave. I was referred to one of his colleagues who practiced in the same office. I hesitated, because I'd felt a bond with the first neurologist; he listened with compassion and was actively interested in my case. A new doctor meant I would have to start over, and I was already pretty low after the spinal tap experience. In the face of an indeterminate delay, though, I decided to schedule an appointment with one of his colleagues.

When I arrived for my appointment, the waiting room was packed and chaotic. Clearly the absence of my original doctor had stretched the capacity of the remaining practitioners. After a moderate wait, I was ushered into one of the examining rooms. A few minutes later, a doctor literally hopped into the room. He had broken his leg the day before and was sporting a new white cast from the tip of his toe to the top of his leg. He was so busy he could not even take time to get crutches. He was swamped with additional patients, in pain, and trying to cope as best he could. I described my previous meetings with his colleague, the battery of tests over the summer, and the recent spinal tap. When I finished speaking, he stared at me blankly. Everything about him said "What do you expect me to do about it, lady?" He was either unable or unwilling to offer any advice about next steps. He was caught up in his own problems. Just like that I discovered that I was walking down a blind alley and had hit the wall. After three months of test after test, culminating in that terrible spinal tap, I was exactly nowhere.

The sense of being exactly nowhere after all this effort sent me into hiding for a number of months. I simply didn't have the energy to go out and find someone new, tell my story again, and take a bunch of tests and be disappointed again. I needed to gather some strength, and the only way I knew to do that was to take a break from pursuit of a diagnosis.

Over the next three months I kept seeing my naturopath faithfully, but I did not pursue any additional medical avenues. This was the start of a pattern repeated over and over in my continuing search for a diagnosis and throughout efforts to treat my illness. I called it the cycle of frustration–action–hope–despair.

The first stage, frustration, was generally what got me restarted seeking a diagnosis. I ignored the illness for as long as I could, then a period of strong symptoms motivated me to take a new step. I'd feel so bad for a stretch of days that I would be forced to realize it was not constructive to ignore the situation any longer. I was frustrated the sickness was dragging on for so long, disappointed at my body's inability to heal itself, and more than a little humiliated by my meager efforts to correct the problem. I told myself—"Enough! Get going and solve this problem." Often, Shelly anticipated these waves of frustration. In some ways he was more sensitive to the symptoms than I was; he saw the effects more objectively.

Shelly: It was a hugely difficult time. Sue was so very exhausted after only a few hours every day, and most often, exhausted even at the very start of the day after hours of recovery sleep. Imagine how much energy it takes to walk on a tightrope, trying to keep your balance. That's what she was doing all day long, and her nights were rolling as if on a boat. As the day wore on a discoloration would grow, larger and darker, under her eyes. They were almost as large and dark as the black smudges painted on under the eyes of football players to cut the glare of the sun. You could just about tell the time of day with them. They were immediately obvious to anyone looking at her. But she wasn't aware of them and the story they were telling, not unless she looked at herself in the mirror every hour, and that's definitely not who she is. Sometimes they would be gone after a long night's sleep. But it most often took longer than that, and after awhile they just built up and were never completely erased during the rest time she had for recovery.

She felt a duty to her workplace; to bring it through this once-in-the-history-of-the-industry transition, and to keep it a "high performance" organization, and an obligation, to the people who worked there, to make the most thoughtful, analytically solid decisions.

When she came up for air she'd realize how terrible she felt, and realize she had to take action to resolve her condition. And we would start down the road again in the search for someone who could offer a diagnosis. We weren't even thinking cure anymore by that point. No sense getting that far ahead. We were just trying to figure out what was wrong!

I remember hiking in the woods in Vermont. You head down a rutted road or a cow path trail into a forest that used to be a field a hundred years ago and eventually, sometimes quickly, sometimes after quite awhile, the trail just peters out and ends. The sugar house that was there is rotted out and gone or the farmhouse was demolished or moved. There is nothing at the end of the trail except perhaps a few trees a little younger than the ones right around them that hints that this was once an intended destination. But there is no "there" there anymore.

That's what this search reminded me of. She would get all the way down the road. And there was nothing there. It wasn't her intended destination. And then she had to turn around and go back to where she started, and start out again in another direction. The effort and anticipation to get there was great. The disappointment at finding nothing was very great. And then she would have to trudge all the way back down that hill. It took time to slowly get through decompression. She'd shift focus back to work. Only after a long enough time could she start out on the search once again.

Once I took action again, I felt hopeful. Making the appointments, telling my story, and hearing ideas for treatment or diagnosis lifted my spirits. It was as if, in hearing my story, the latest medical adviser took some of the responsibility to make progress off my shoulders. My confidence was further bolstered when there were new ideas about the cause of the symptoms and new suggestions for treatment. The prescription worked as long as it remained uncertain whether the ideas were failing yet again. The downside of this stage was that it was followed, too closely, by despair. When a test failed to identify a diagnosis, or the treatments failed, I was emotionally devastated. Whether that was due to the emotional incontinence of the illness or not, I still felt miserable.

After a disappointing diagnosis cycle, I was not able to start the steep climb back to renewed hope immediately. I needed to rest and recuperate emotionally before trying something new. This rest and recuperation continued until I regained sufficient energy to be frustrated, then the cycle would begin again. After my neurologist stopped working (to deal with his own illness) I went into a three-month period of rest from the emotional roller coaster of seeking a diagnosis.

✳   ✳   ✳

I looked like a raccoon, with dark circles under each eye, and I walked at a slant, often reaching out to touch the wall for aid. People who knew me recognized I was not my normal self. Almost weekly, someone suggested a physician to see, a new diet, nutritional supplements, books I should read. I kept a loosely organized list of these suggestions, noting in particular those entries mentioned by more than one person. The kindness of these people, who braved their hesitation about approaching someone sick and offering some advice, was an unanticipated gift. Even though it often embarrassed me, particularly because I still questioned whether I was really sick, I was very grateful. Like finding the first neurologist after my friend Jacob offered help, these offerings often directed me to the right next step.

Now, though, after eight long months of illness, I began to have my first serious doubts that I could both get well and continue to work, even at my reduced pace. It was awkward to discuss the idea of leaving work with any of my colleagues. I sought out a consultant, Jesse, who worked closely with the executive team. Jesse knew me well and knew the challenges Bonneville Power Administration faced with the latest reorganization and the changing regulatory climate.

The reorganization planned in the spring of 1996 was phased in over the summer and the early fall. The time right after a reorganization is very delicate. I was aware of the strain the reorganization placed on employees, strain added to their existing fears about deregulation and job security. It was a fragile period, and the success of the reorganization depended on how well we navigated these tricky next few months.

Jesse and I took a long walk in the woods, and she helped me focus my thoughts and feelings about remaining at work. I kept coming back to my desire to work long enough to ensure that the benefits of the reorganization were realized. Other executives were buried in detailed planning, but I worked on systems that measured the overall results. I wanted to stay and work in order to give others some experience with the new systems, to work out the inevitable problems and see for myself whether these ideas would prove to be the solutions I'd deeply felt they could be. I needed that much closure for this surprise ending of my career. At the same time, I questioned whether, when the time came, I would just move the goal line and seek additional closure on the next set of challenges. There was no way to be sure, but the walk and the conversation provided a focused agenda for the next six to nine months.

In early September of 1996 I'd initiated an employee meeting every Monday morning to discuss issues of concern to employees about the newly completed reorganization. The meetings were open to all employees; we even had phone connections to remote locations. Fifty to one hundred people usually attended—a large enough number to spread the word. I started off the meeting with a short ten-minute talk and then hoped some employee, either in the room or on the phone connection, would be brave enough to share the latest horrific rumor. Most of the time I was able to give the facts behind the rumor and dispel some concerns. In each case, I benefited from hearing what employees were hearing.

A side benefit of these meetings was the inspiring conversations I had with others who were sick. People frequently sought me out after these sessions, in the halls and in the cafeteria, to share their health challenges. It was rather uncomfortable when several people who had multiple sclerosis, the condition I had recently ruled out, shared their diagnosis. Often these people were secretive about their conditions, concerned that illness would limit their chances for advancement if it were widely known. I felt a personal connection to these coworkers and their stories and privileged that they chose to share them with me. I was surprised at the wellspring of empathy and compassion. Before I was sick myself I would have thought chronically sick people would be self-pitying or complaining. Although there certainly were those elements in some individuals, much more often I saw and felt courage and compassion from them.

I kept up my forty-hour work-week schedule all fall and ignored my condition as best I could. By December, ignoring the problem was not the solution.

December 11, 1996

I have had a couple of tough weeks—off balance, morning nausea, achy, very tired. Today I feel the same, and depressed. I am just so tired all the time. I do keep going—I have only missed my 3 miles of walking each day a few times. It seems to get my equilibrium going. But my joints are aching, particularly my hips, and the abdominal pain is back. I have a rash on my right hip that won't go away. My spine has itched since the spinal tap.

I seem to function okay mentally but I am emotionally over-sensitive or else totally flat. But I also have doubts that I do feel poorly—maybe I have never felt any better. There is this guilt that perhaps I am attached to this illness, dependent on it in some way. I still see that I am better—not deaf, less actively dizzy, more energy sometimes—but for the last two weeks. But I guess this is what happens, it isn't linear, there is no straight line progress—no diagnosis, no treatment, no cure . . . no illness?

I am very grateful for what is sustaining me. Shelly, his love and support is miraculous. The neighborhood walks and friendly faces. Bunkee, she makes me smile and gets me outside. My vastly slower pace at work has made for better relationships and perspective. I have reflected, I have sat and read, I have rested. I have spent hours alone thinking and meditating.

There are no conclusions, it is not over. I just wanted a record, a snapshot.

There was a small bright side: A new quality to my life was emerging. I spent more time sitting and reading. I was becoming a fixture in my neighborhood; you could tell time by seeing me walk past with my energetic young dog, Bunkee. Her antics were one of the few things that could reliably make me laugh. I was forming casual relationships with the neighbors I passed on our walks. These small things and the slower pace were beginning to restore some small measure of balance in my life.

Life fell into a pattern of surviving the work week and recovering on the weekend. This pattern wasn't disrupted until January, when two events caused my frustration to resurface and begin the cycle again. First, my naturopath told me he was out of approaches to try; he knew he wasn't helping, and couldn't help. At the same time, I started to have problems with my memory—another alarming symptom.

I was still sick. I still didn't have a diagnosis. I didn't even have a doctor. I was still frustrated. I didn't know what the new year would hold. But I absolutely knew I had to do something.

Speaking From Experience: Tips to Make Your Journey Easier

1. The visual migraines and skin rashes were my only new symptoms during this period. However, nine months of constant, debilitating symptoms took a physical as well as an emotional toll. Although it sounds absurd to say I wasn't sure I was sick, there is real power in

having a diagnosis. In contrast, there is strong self-doubt and confusion when no medical professional you locate can diagnose your illness. Unfortunately, this is typical for vestibular disorders. If you think you have a vestibular disorder, seek out a specialist.

2. The aftermath of the spinal tap forced me to see that a lifelong approach I had to problems—to try harder and harder, to expend more and more energy—was no longer working for me. This was the first fundamental change I made to accommodate the new person I had become. I found that many of my "well person" strategies for living did not translate well into my new "sick person" life. There's no doubt you will trip over a few of these as well—in the end, they are powerful learning experiences.

3. I also saw the first glimmer of benefits from a slower pace, even though it was forced on me by sickness. It was essential to embrace these moments of strolling rather than running, chatting with a neighbor, or petting my dog, because they were the areas in my life where I received more energy than I invested. Watch yourself closely and identify your sources of personal energy.

4

The Medical Fog Clears

JANUARY 1997–MAY 1997

The cycle of frustration–action–hope–despair moved from the frustration at year's end to action when I decided to pursue a lead I'd discovered in *Osler's Web* by Hillary Johnson. I'd read the book the preceding summer. It had detailed descriptions of the history of chronic fatigue syndrome (CFS), symptoms, and the scientific research currently being conducted. I was relieved to find lists of symptoms identical to mine, yet it sounded like the CFS patients were far more debilitated. I returned to the book each time I had a new symptom and was somewhat comforted to find it listed as well. *Osler's Web* also gave me an appreciation for the difficulty of finding a physician capable of treating CFS because it was such a new and somewhat controversial diagnosis. In fact this was one of the more hopeless aspects of chronic fatigue: No one appeared to know how to treat it. In some ways this was worse than having no diagnosis at all.

I became fixated on seeing Dr. Mark Loveless, the Portland (Oregon) physician mentioned several times in the book. I was not convinced I had CFS, but I needed to test my opinion, and he was my only lead at the moment. I was sick and tired and not very hopeful, and I didn't really expect a conclusive final answer anymore. I just wanted to do everything I could. If I really had CFS then I wanted to hear it from someone who truly knew what CFS was. If the accurate diagnosis of my illness was going to be achieved by the process of elimination, I had to pursue this lead.

Dr. Loveless was a physician at Oregon Health Sciences University who taught at the university and staffed a clinic for AIDS and CFS patients. He was involved with CFS because of its similarities to AIDS. I was intimidated by his credentials, particularly because I still doubted the severity of my condition. Before calling for the appointment, I called Bruce, one of my neighbors who was also a physician and a professor at Oregon Health Sciences University, to reassure myself I was pursuing a reasonable path. He and his physician wife, Ora, frequently stopped me on my walks to inquire how I was doing, so he was generally familiar with my situation. Bruce thought Dr. Loveless was a logical next step and offered to assist me in quickly confirming an appointment in Loveless's very busy schedule. This was the push I needed.

I made notes to prepare for my upcoming appointment so I was able to present as accurate a description of symptoms as possible.

March 13, 1997

On bad days I experience muscle and joint aching, stomach cramps, skin rashes and herpes outbreaks, headaches, heart palpitations, depression, "emotional incontinence." I have developed vision problems including light sensitivity and scotoma or flashing lights that block patches of vision. On very bad days the room might spin, move back and forth or I might have discomfort walking while moving my head even a little.

I also told him about symptoms that now were a constant daily pattern: ear ringing, the final remnant of the early deafness; nausea, particularly in the morning; lack of balance, including problems with depth perception, "things moving inside my head"; and things appearing to move away from me. I also described how I forced myself to get up in the morning and how I never had any energy even to talk or interact socially. I described the onset of symptoms as associated with a virus.

After hearing my story, Dr. Loveless became quite animated. He swiveled quickly to the large whiteboard in the office; stood up, nearly knocking over a stack of papers on his desk; grabbed two different colored markers; and began to draw pictures on the board to explain what was going on in my body. He indicated that I did have CFS but explained that this was not a complete diagnosis, especially in my case. It was his theory that CFS was a result of a wide variety of disease processes culminating in too much input to the brain.

In my case, Dr. Loveless thought the root cause of the problems was one or both of my ears. He described the situation from the perspective of my brain: My balance was off and my brain was getting conflicting signals from my right and left ears. As my brain worked to keep me upright, it sent "alerts" to my heart, eyes, muscles, and joints. Because of the unrelenting alerts, my entire system was under stress—on alert—for more than a year.

No wonder I was exhausted! This explained the heart palpitations, the vision problems, and the sore muscles and aching joints. He even had a theory for the mysterious skin rashes I recently developed.

Finally, finally! A diagnosis that could explain the entire set of symptoms! They were all connected! This was a huge moment! I would have danced with joy but I was of course . . . exhausted.

Dr. Loveless strongly recommended I avoid increased fatigue over the course of each week. He emphasized that I needed a routine to conserve energy rather than use every ounce of energy I could muster. In his experience the only way to reverse the fatigue was to "get my activity level below my energy level."

This simple statement contained so much wisdom. Years later it would become my mantra. On this first day, it merely sounded impossible. He also told me I might not be able to both work, and get well.

My fear about getting my hopes up only to be let down again vanished. Dr. Loveless understood my symptoms and clearly described what caused them. He wasn't intimidating; he was a normal human being, a friend of my friends. My fear of being dismissed by him was completely unfounded. I had allowed myself to be a victim, to believe medical professionals were unapproachable and too important to worry themselves with my small concerns.

I had to learn this lesson many times: Positive rewards came whenever I pursued my health issues with the same professional approach I used in the rest of my life.

Dr. Loveless referred me to Dr. Owen Black, an oto-neurologist who specialized in vestibular, or balance, disorders. Dr. Loveless held Dr. Black in high regard because of Dr. Black's consistent success in diagnosing and treating a wide variety of vestibular problems.

This was the first time I'd ever heard the word *vestibular*. *Vestibular* refers to the parts of the ear that contribute to balance. Dr. Black was a leading physician and a researcher who had created diagnostic tests and treatment protocols for a range of balance disorders. I later learned he was involved with NASA, conducting research on the effects of weightlessness on balance. This was more than I had hoped for. I now had a better understanding of CFS, I knew there was an additional factor complicating my condition, and the expert who might help was right in town! I also made a follow-up appointment with Dr. Loveless, who committed to work with Dr. Black to identify the cause of my problems.

I arrived at Dr. Black's office for my first appointment and immediately noticed a difference right in the waiting room: The lights were low and it was quiet. The receptionist gave me the usual insurance forms to fill out, but in addition she handed me a checklist of symptoms: *balance, vertigo, dizziness, hearing loss, tinnitus, pressure in ears, ear pain, nausea, visual sensitivity, headache*, and *noise sensitivity*. Simply reading the list made me cry with relief. I was overwhelmed with a feeling of coming home, a sense I could relax and stop pushing so hard for clarity. This was a place where other people knew what I was going through. I had every symptom on the list! The severity rating scale was from one to ten; one represented normalcy, no symptom, and ten represented a disabling symptom level. For the first time in months and months I was with people who recognized my symptoms and might really know what caused them.

Dr. Black personally came to the door, called my name, and escorted me to the treatment room. This was his custom; I'd never seen it with any other doctor before or since. He took a detailed history of my illness and asked several interesting questions about my family members, such as whether either of my parents had prematurely white hair. The next step was a series of balance tests to be administered over the next month. The test results would give him a basis for making a diagnosis and initiating treatment. More tests! I wasn't impatient with more tests, though; for the first time, they were being ordered by a professional within a specific specialty who would understand what to do with the results. This was the point where the search for a diagnosis had finally stopped being a process of elimination.

Dr. Black also reassured me about emotions and mental function. I was very worried about this because of upcoming testimony I had to give in a work-related lawsuit.

Dr. Black explained that the brain puts a higher priority on "executive functions" when there is a stress. Balance, like breathing, heartbeat, and the other circulatory activities, is an executive function. Short-term memory and emotional control are not executive functions.

To further comfort me he showed me a long list of scientific studies documenting that memory and emotion are affected by vestibular problems. When the balance issues were under control, my brain could stop overworking on balance and return to other, more normal functions. It was likely my memory would return to normal. This was good news!

When the balance issues were under control, my brain could stop overworking on balance and return to other more normal functions. It was likely my memory would return to normal.

Over the next several weeks I completed a variety of diagnostic tests. Several of the tests were done as I stood on a platform surrounded by high walls on three sides. The floor as well as the walls moved around while I tried to keep my balance as best I could. I was trussed up in a harness so I couldn't hurt myself if (when!) I fell. For some tests a probe with a tiny balloon was inflated into each of my ears to simulate pressure increases while the platform moved. In other tests, I was blindfolded and tried to balance without any visual cues while the floor moved. I didn't even know what we were measuring, but I was impressed with the equipment and the computer interface. I wanted to get an "A," but I didn't even know what an "A" was!

Other tests required that electrodes be attached to my forehead as I watched objects while turning my head. This series of tests, which involved head and eye movements, was most disturbing. At one point I was strapped into a chair that rotated while lights were projected on the circular walls. The technician instructed "Tell me a girl's name starting with "A," and then "Starting with a "B," and so on down the alphabet. I was shocked at how difficult it was. This engaged my brain and kept me from zoning out on the dots projected on the revolving walls. I had to concentrate. I did, but the engagement certainly didn't keep me from becoming nauseated and calling a halt to the test.

Every test was repeated several times and my responses measured and recorded. The purpose of the tests was to cause symptoms that could then be measured in order to pinpoint the cause of the problem. I went into each session more or less normal and left severely dizzy and nauseated. Many days I had to rest in the testing area or the waiting room before I was confident I could drive home, even though it was only a mile. The medical staff were unfailing in their caring support—offering tea, encouraging me to rest, and acknowledging how difficult the tests were for all patients. It took me a day or two to recover after each test, but I kept telling myself it was worth it for a diagnosis.

I'd spent a year unsure if I was sick and deeply frustrated by the lack of a diagnosis. These were the first tests—since the rudimentary test given by the neurologist—that consistently produced the symptoms I experienced every day. Even in my fog I knew this was good news, that these were the right tests and that ultimately they would define my problem. I had high hopes these tests would lead to a diagnosis.

The tests were intellectually interesting because each variation provided some different piece of data and revealed information about brain and balance function that I took completely for granted. I was able to engage my brain to observe the procedures and the data, but I was emotionally flat and lifeless, incapable of expressing interest or enthusiasm. This was consistent with how I felt in my broader life, but somehow it was more apparent in this different environment. It was as if there were a wall between the rest of the world and me—like one of those protective shields from the old tooth decay commercials. I could see things going on, but I felt no response and had no emotional energy to connect with them. When I was not flat and emotionless I was bursting into tears for no apparent reason. That mattered less here, because Dr. Black's staff accepted it as a normal response to the stress of the tests.

A week after the last test I had my second appointment with Dr. Black to hear the results. He said my problem was definitely vestibular. However, on the basis of the results of the tests and the history I provided, he was not able to determine why the problem was occurring or what the cause was. I exhibited symptoms from several problems. The symptoms conflicted or overlapped and made the diagnosis hard to differentiate, and that might mean there were multiple causes. He needed to determine the main problem and work from there. He wanted me to come back in six months and take some of the tests again because he thought the results would be different at a later point. He said he frequently observed fluctuation and unpredictable results when a patient's condition is active or ongoing.

So long, hope, here's our old friend despair again. I'd been so convinced I would hear a definitive diagnosis. Dr. Black's suggestion sounded very logical, but it was also incomplete. Six months sounded like an eternity. I asked why it was taking so long when I'd already wandered around for more than a year seeking a diagnosis. I was humbled when he told me one year was very rapid; many patients he treated took four to six years to be referred to his office. I left his office in stunned silence. It wasn't a dead end; I now knew I had vestibular problems. On the other hand, it certainly was not the breakthrough I'd hoped for in the search for a diagnosis.

Fortunately, I was still seeing Dr. Loveless each month for CFS, so I at least had a next step and was not immobilized by the despair. Before my next appointment with him Dr. Loveless spoke with Dr. Black. Dr. Loveless told me they were both convinced the source of my problems was the vestibular system. Dr. Black's testing had located the source of the problem. For some reason the brain signals from my eyes and muscles were being distorted or interrupted by information from my ears. There were several possible causes, and I exhibited symptoms of each one, so it was not possible to provide a further diagnosis, or to begin a treatment, at this early point. Because we had a six-month hiatus in further diagnostic progress, Dr. Loveless recommended trying a month with no symptoms to see if we could reduce the fatigue. This meant medicating all the symptoms. With six months to wait and a job I still needed to perform, it seemed like the right next step.

> Brain signals from my eyes and muscles were being distorted or interrupted by information from my ears.

Shelly accompanied me on this visit both to provide moral support and to better understand my condition. He asked several questions I was not focused enough to think of. At each doctor's visit, I went in with a list of questions and got clear answers to those questions, but if additional issues came up in the discussion I was able to ask and absorb only about half of the answers. I'd begun to keep notes of each doctor visit for later reference because I frequently forgot or got confused about some symptom. There were a lot of symptoms to keep track of and, right now, my memory was not entirely reliable.

When Shelly first offered to go with me to my appointment, I resisted. I felt silly and childlike, needing help to get to the doctor. But he insisted, and I understood his point. This illness affected his life almost as much as mine, and he deserved first-hand information. After more than a year of illness, I needed to admit this was not the typical medical interaction. It was taking all the skills and insight we both could muster. He was my partner, my confidant, and my best friend. After meeting Dr. Loveless, Shelly was better able to observe my reactions and give positive suggestions. He provided a different perspective on the illness, and he observed things I missed.

> *Shelly:* The most important thing I learned in three and a half years of graduate school at MIT was a deceptively simple statement in a statistics seminar: "Half of all doctors are above average, which means the other half are below." Sue had found a doctor who was so clearly above average. This guy finally had a lead! The first real one we had heard in over a year of searching!

This series of doctors' visits, this chapter in the search for a diagnosis, was not a total disappointment; neither was it an unqualified success. I did not feel as desperate as I had earlier; I was confident about the medical team advising me. I had gotten to the right specialty even if the advice had not yet crystallized into a clear diagnosis. On the other hand, I was not filled with hope for near-term clarity. I was uncomfortably suspended between both poles. I continued to struggle at work. The transformation back and forth from being a sick, emotionally incontinent person who cried at the slightest provocation to assuming the posture of a leader who was calm in the face of challenges and problems was taking a toll.

The greatest benefit of this phase in the search for a diagnosis was that I was finally convinced I was indeed sick. There was now a series of tests that showed something was wrong. The "something wrong" simply did not have a name—yet.

Speaking From Experience: Tips to Make Your Journey Easier

1. My symptom tracking finally paid dividends as useful information for both Dr. Loveless and Dr. Black. It was helpful to be able to present both "normal" day symptoms and "bad" day symptoms. Both doctors were readily able to interpret and explain the symptoms as part of an underlying vestibular problem. This gave me confidence about the diagnosis because no other doctor had described an underlying problem that addressed all my symptoms.

2. I brought notes as well as a list of questions to every medical appointment and took detailed notes of the responses and explanations. Despite this, there was more information than I was able to comprehend and record. Perhaps it was the illness; regardless of the reason, I recognized I needed help. One of the most positive steps I took in my long journey toward a diagnosis was to ask my husband to accompany me to these medical appointments. I needed a partner to be sure I didn't miss something important, and he needed direct contact with the professionals who were providing explanations and advice. Do yourself a favor and take a partner or a friend to your medical appointments.

3. The long time frame for diagnosis of vestibular problems was beyond my ability to comprehend. I was only able to see maybe the next six months. It never dawned on me that the long time frame for diagnosis would persist into future diagnoses and treatments. I still wanted the instant cure. Diagnosis begins the treatment stage—it's a big positive step, but it's not a cure.

4. Dr. Loveless provided some invaluable advice, some genuine wisdom: Keep your activity level below your energy level. In other words, don't get tired. This sounds deceptively simple but proved difficult to achieve. I started by limiting activities—trying to identify things that made me feel worse and avoiding them. I also simply did fewer things. Even though I believed this advice was temporary, until I got well, I felt I was losing parts of myself when I curtailed activity. I tried to follow this advice for years and years, with little success, but I kept coming back to it when I experienced my worst symptoms. It worked, if only I could figure out how to live it. Take this advice to heart: Keep your activity level below your energy level.

Suggested Reading

Johnson, H. (1996). *Osler's Web: Inside the Labyrinth of the Chronic Fatigue Syndrome Epidemic*. New York: Crown Publishers.

5

The Surprise End of a Satisfying Career

JUNE 1997–OCTOBER 1997

I was having memory problems. I had first noticed it in January 1997. I began to forget small things and could no longer keep track of my crowded and ever-changing calendar. Because I always wrote down lists of tasks, kept good notes, and prepared for every meeting, I was able to control the problems these memory lapses caused. However, I was more and more aware of them and they began to shake my confidence.

I needed to retain and use hundreds of facts to do my job effectively, ranging from simple facts, like when meetings were scheduled and whom should attend, to key pieces of data that would help determine the overall strategy to address a specific issue. Frequently, I was the leader of decision-making discussions, and my grasp of relevant facts was an essential tool to focus the discussion and highlight the major issues.

My increasing difficulties with short-term memory were very apparent when I was slated to be a key witness in an upcoming arbitration. In my previous position as the executive in charge of the Energy Resources division I'd authorized the purchase of a power plant. The 1994 marketing strategy concluded that this power plant was no longer needed because the Bonneville Power Administration (BPA) was losing customers and didn't need additional power plants. In several similar cases BPA had terminated plants and reached a financial agreement with the plant owner. In this case there was no agreement and the plant owners filed suit for more than $1 billions in damages. It was an extremely significant proceeding for both parties.

In cases of this magnitude, BPA was supported by attorneys from the Department of Justice rather than our own legal staff. The attorneys had begun preliminary preparation and interviews in early January. They were developing a strategy for the case, figuring out who should provide which pieces of testimony and assessing the strengths and weaknesses of various witnesses. After two interviews two weeks apart, I could not recall the basics of the case or even what we discussed two weeks earlier. Throughout my academic life and my career, I had relied heavily on my almost-photographic short-term memory. Still, I knew this challenge was an order of magnitude greater because of my illness. I set aside twice as much time to prepare and planned to focus all my attention on the case when the time arrived.

Over the next few months I worked with my attorney regularly but was not making noticeable progress remembering the facts of my role in the case. I needed to study voluminous notes and memoranda about the decision to purchase the plant. Then I needed to put them in context with the other events occurring in the industry. It was important to recall the three-year chronology and be able to answer questions about the rationale and facts relevant to the key decisions. When I'd had to testify for cases like this in the past I simply went over the relevant information a few times until I was fully prepared. This time these pieces were not falling into place.

I decided to take a few weeks off from my regular daily tasks and spend my full time reading, rereading, and drilling myself on the relevant information. I had to reduce the other work requirements on my brain to free up space over and above the executive function requirements Dr. Black had described to me. On the basis of our extensive interviews, my attorney drafted a general outline of the testimony I needed to provide as well as a general idea of the type of questions I might face. I went over and over and over this information until I was confident I could present the quality of testimony required. About two days before I was scheduled to testify, the information clicked into focus. Just in the nick of time!

The arbitration itself was in Denver, Colorado. I arrived late in the afternoon before I was due to appear in court. I went to the arbitration site just to get a feel for the layout of the room, where the witness sat, and how the attorneys and arbitrators interacted—anything to make me a little more comfortable. All the participants were aware I was having health difficulties, but because my diagnosis was still being refined I wasn't able to request any specific changes or accommodation that would make the situation easier. I could request a break at any time, but I wasn't sure whether it would be better just to press on through and finish the testimony as quickly as possible. I was concerned an extended rest period might erase my fragile memory banks. I went over the testimony with my attorney the evening before the hearing. I remembered the events in the right order and recalled all the major issues. He seemed relieved.

I knew I needed to be well rested for the ordeal, so I went to bed early the night before and went right to sleep. Of course the hotel fire alarm went off at 3:00 a.m., complete with flashing strobe lights and sirens! I bounded out of my ninth-floor bed, heart pounding. It was quickly confirmed as a false alarm but I couldn't get back to sleep and spent hours fueling my anxiety about the upcoming events. Shaky and anxious, I met with my attorney for breakfast to confirm last-minute details and then headed for the arbitration.

First, I presented my direct testimony. This was very much like a dance performance. My attorney asked questions and I was able to answer them based on all the information I'd prepared ahead of time. There were no surprises, no missteps during our formal dance. Then the opposing attorney asked me a series of questions. I had to listen intently to these questions and discern where the attorney was trying to lead me, what point he was trying to make. If I could do that, I would be able to develop a thoughtful response to support the case my utility was making.

I was on the witness stand for a day and a half. There were times I wasn't sure I would make it, but the all-consuming focus on the questions and responses kept me from thinking about how I felt physically. It was back to adrenaline and my old mode of pushing through. It took enormous energy to get through this, but I did.

My attorney had been concerned about whether I could provide solid testimony right up to the last minute. He'd consistently heard positive reports from all my colleagues about my ability to testify and communicate, but he hadn't worked with me before and hadn't seen much of that during our preparations. He saw me struggling to recall minor facts and never able to put the larger picture together. Now he was overjoyed I'd managed to get through this successfully. I was, too!

My jubilation was short lived. The adrenaline began to dissipate immediately. During the cab ride to the airport I realized I was totally exhausted. Once I checked in for my flight I decided to get something to eat, hoping food would boost my energy. I found a cozy restaurant in a quiet corner near my gate and ordered a bowl of soup. I was nauseous after only a few spoonfuls and started feeling a warm flush. I paid my bill and rushed to the restroom to avoid throwing up in the restaurant.

I was slightly panicked as I sat at the gate waiting to board my flight. What if I was going to throw up the whole way? Should I stay in Denver until I felt steadier, or should I make the huge physical effort to get home? There was no real choice, though; I wanted to get home.

By the time I got on the plane I was in a full-fledged episode: muscles aching, migraine, and nausea; the room spun; and I had no energy. I started to meditate the instant I got settled into my seat, and I didn't stop for the full two-hour flight. Every ounce of calm from the meditation went into easing my panic and controlling the nausea. By the time I landed I was so exhausted I was disoriented.

I called Shelly from the airport in Portland, and he came to pick me up. I could barely speak. Everything swirled around me on the ride home. Shelly had never seen me this sick before. As I rode back wrapped in exhausted silence he asked me every few minutes if I was okay. All I could do was nod. Later on he told me that he had started to think about which hospital emergency room he should take me to. There were three we passed on the ride home. As we passed each one he decided to wait for the next one, to see if my responses were more animated. It took a week of rest before I was able to return to work.

This was the first dramatic illustration of a scenario that would occur again and again. I found reserves of energy and concentration to perform when it was a priority. Afterward, I had a significant relapse and strong out-of-balance symptoms. It was the exact opposite of Dr. Loveless's sage advice to keep my activity level below my energy level. At stressful or particularly busy times, my activity level exceeded my energy level by so much that I was thrown into a serious downward spiral for a week. Years later I began to understand the physical impact of these stressful situations on my balance system. In these early months it was confusing to be able to rise to an occasion and, as soon as the pressure was off, to crash.

The Denver trip was a stark illustration of the extent to which my work depleted my energy. If I'd wondered about that correlation before, there was no doubt now. After I rested enough to return to work I renewed my efforts to reduce my schedule and conserve my energy. I now worked thirty to thirty-five hours a week, came in late and left early. I'd already stopped bringing work home earlier in the year because I was consistently too exhausted to complete it anyway. I started to worry I was hurting the utility because I couldn't dedicate enough time to my job to do it well.

During our June appointment Dr. Loveless was disturbed to hear about the effects of the Denver trip. On the positive side, he was pleased that the symptom suppression medications relieved the bulk of my symptoms during normal times. On most days I was now only nauseated with a headache and experiencing slight movement or imbalance. He repeated his admonition to keep my activity level below my energy level, something I'd thus far been unable to achieve. He told me if I was able to keep my activity level low enough so that I did not get tired the symptoms might subside over the course of a year. He also warned me that the reverse applied as well; he was not optimistic I would get better if I could not reduce my activity level. I resolved to stick to my reduced work schedule more consistently.

It was very painful to face the fact that I might not be able to both work and get well, that I couldn't get my activity level low enough if I were working. I began to explore the possibility of a disability retirement, just exploring—not starting—the process. I was still hoping that after my six-month follow up appointment with Dr. Black there would be a diagnosis, a treatment regimen, and a fast recovery. I wanted to get well; I wanted to keep working. But I felt so poorly I realized I needed to follow Dr. Loveless's advice—now.

Just as I was getting used to the idea of stopping work, my boss informed me he intended to leave in September. We worked together closely, and he was concerned about my plans given my health problems. We decided it would be best for the organization if I stayed on after his departure, perhaps until his permanent replacement was named. I was responsible for the internal operations of the utility, whereas he focused his attention on customer and political issues. By remaining after his departure, I could provide needed stability (the irony of providing stability in my "unbalanced state" would have amused me had I not been too exhausted to see the humor). I was still uncertain about the feasibility of a disability retirement and what I really wanted to do was get well and stay.

I certainly wanted to stay at BPA long enough to see measurable results for the professional goals I'd defined on my walk in the woods with Jesse the previous fall. Seeing those goals through to the end meant staying at work at least through October 1997, when fiscal year annual performance reviews were completed. Setting a target retirement date of February 1998 would allow me to finish my work and provide a smooth transition to new leadership. I started the summer of 1997 resolving to work through February 1998.

It was satisfying to see others take hold of the systems I envisioned and improve them significantly so they met the needs of the new organizations. I was also pleased with the progress on setting and measuring results, meaningful results linked to long-term strategy. Many of the new organizations had shown a great deal of creativity and initiative to identify the best results on which to focus; develop efficient measurement systems; and perhaps most important, to turn employees loose to figure out how to achieve the results.

With all the projects at work percolating along on schedule, it seemed perfect timing for my and Shelly's summer vacation. I also needed a break from work to get a clearer picture of how I was really doing.

Anne, my sister who had accompanied me on the Alzheimer's facility search for my father, had moved to London the previous fall, and we now planned a visit for early July. Shelly and I flew to London and spent a few days there before driving to the Cotswolds for some walking. This was the perfect vacation for me in my current condition: It was cool, the schedule was flexible, and the walking was therapeutic. Even though I got tired, there was ample opportunity to rest. As long as we were in the countryside I felt quite normal. Being in London was another story. We went to the famous boat races at Henley-on-Thames. A large crowd was packed along both sides of the riverbank, and all the nausea, imbalance, and fatigue came rushing back. This was one of the first times I realized that crowds or events with a lot of people milling around were a problem.

Anne was an epidemiologist. Epidemiologists are trained to be very observant, and Anne was indeed a good one. She was increasingly frustrated with my lack of progress with the illness. She openly blamed my work pressures. For many years she'd viewed my dedication to work as obsessive and felt I took too much responsibility for the state of affairs at my job. She did not think I was taking my medical condition seriously enough. She strongly doubted I would be able to continue to work, and she also despaired I would ever be able to let go and resign. Because she never hesitated to speak her mind, I knew all this, and I knew that she was worried about me to the point of being angry with me. But I was too tired and numb to react, and I certainly did not thank her for her concern.

From London we flew to Nice to meet friends in the south of France. They had made the arrangements, and we stayed in the tower of a lovely manor house. What we didn't count on was the heat. I dragged myself through a long list of enchanting places only by brute force and collapsed at the end of each day. The mornings were best because they were coolest. By early afternoon it was roasting and I was nauseated and dizzy. Our friends were clearly worried about me, and I was sorry to ruin their vacation. They were good sports about our limited ability to explore the surroundings and very solicitous of my ability to join in. I felt like an unwelcome speed bump on the highway of our good times—again.

All of the lectures and concern from the people close to me were making an impression. They saw how different I was from the person they used to know. Somewhere along the way, I'd lost track of how I used to feel.

It sounds preposterous to say, "I forgot how I felt when I was well," but it was the truth. Sickness had become my reality. As I lived each day with the nausea, dizziness, headaches, and other symptoms, they began to be the norm. I had imagined chronic illness as deeply sad—dramatic, if not tragic. My own experience wasn't dramatic at all; it was unrelenting, but there was no high drama, no tragedy. Maybe the lack of emotion was a key. I felt emotionally flat all the time. I was used to having boundless energy and enthusiasm, but now they were gone. I was so tired I barely noticed. On the surface my life was what it had always been: the same job, the same family, the same house, the same interests. It took more out of me to do less. I couldn't keep up anymore. I remembered being tired before, but had I been this tired?

✳   ✳   ✳

The failed vacation to England and France was a stark reminder of how far my condition had deteriorated. The symptoms had not gone away for a year and a half and counting. Only the early deafness was gone; all the other symptoms were still present, and the list appeared to get longer and longer. When I stepped outside my normal routine I was able to see my limitations more clearly. My friends and family were not hesitant about pointing them out either. I faced the new reality: I decided to apply for a disability retirement.

Applying for the disability retirement was a huge emotional hurdle. I still fought my own perceptions that I wasn't really sick. I sometimes felt I was a malingerer trying to dupe people into thinking I was sick. I simply couldn't see that I "deserved" a disability, whatever that meant. The BPA professional who counseled me about the application process saw I was struggling with all these issues. He patiently explained that if I did not deserve the disability, it would not be granted. He approached the issues in a businesslike way. From a business perspective it was a straightforward decision. When one took away all the emotion, it was simply the next logical step. I understood that intellectually, but I still didn't feel it emotionally. Taking disability felt like a defeat. I wasn't used to that.

Disability retirement applications were frequently denied, and even when accepted they usually took at least six months for approval. I needed to fill out a series of forms and request information from several of my doctors, so I decided it was time to get started. By late August I had finished the paperwork. Organizing the application showed me how very many accommodations I had already made to the illness—extensive time off, greatly reduced hours, and no business travel. I didn't tell anyone at work other than my boss about the application for disability retirement. I still thought it was unlikely the application would be approved, and I certainly did not think it would be approved soon.

✳   ✳   ✳

On Tuesday September 23, 1997, just three weeks after I filed the disability application, it was approved. My initial reaction was panic: My boss was leaving in one week, and the letter granting the disability said I had to stop work immediately. I would be leaving at exactly the worst time for the organization instead of making the smooth transition I'd envisioned. I was also overwhelmed that my career was suddenly coming to an end. The reality of working for almost twenty-five years, now confident in my abilities and at peace with my shortcomings, was replaced in very short order by complete uncertainty.

I shared the news of the disability approval with my boss and the colleague designated to serve as his temporary replacement. The three of us put together the pieces of a plan. I would retire in three weeks rather than the immediate departure specified in the approval. These were special circumstances and three weeks provided sufficient time to close out many of my critical activities: year-end reviews, hiring, the orderly transfer of leadership on key projects.

September 27, 1997

I announced to the Executive group that I was leaving yesterday at a strategic planning session. It was quite emotional for me and for others. I care about the institution, the people and their regard for me. Their reaction was a totally uplifting and supportive experience. I do not know when I have felt so validated—and appreciated—I wish I could bottle the feeling. Everyone's main concern was for my health which let me know how evident my sickness was . . . I can't think of a time that I so much needed support and received it so fully.

The next Monday morning I announced my imminent departure to the rest of the organization. I felt a special connection to the group of employees who had accepted my offer to talk and listen each Monday morning, so it seemed like the right place to say goodbye. It wasn't necessary to explain why I was leaving; everyone saw I was sick. Speculation had been mounting about my departure for months. I did want to explain the timing, and I wanted to share with these employees what an honor it was to be a leader of BPA at this moment in history, regardless of the difficulty. Now, though, I needed to give myself a chance to get well.

My schedule was booked solid with appointments to complete interviews, finish performance reviews, delegate projects, and say a few goodbyes. It went by in a blur.

October 15, 1997

My last employee meeting. Jack said some very nice words and people stood up and applauded—my only "standing ovation." It was really moving. I am sleepwalking my way out. I'm too tired—both physically and emotionally—to do this. I am making the right move and I am almost done.

On my last day, I packed up boxes of papers and belongings and carried them to my car in the basement garage. As I went down for the last time, I thought with relief, "I made it out alive."

Speaking From Experience: Tips to Make Your Journey Easier

1. The trial in Denver illustrated an important phenomenon: Sometimes a vestibular patient can perform under pressure, but it will come with a high cost. This pattern repeated itself again and again. Although avoiding the stress is the best alternative, some situations are unavoidable and the only thing you can do is plan for recovery. In my case, this extreme event was an important teacher, a blaring warning signal. My job was filled with similar challenges, and I was not equipped to rise to the challenge on a regular basis. It is tempting to think you will get over the illness and return to normal life. Just in case, keep notes of work as well as life situations that cause significant symptoms and long recovery. These notes will help you make decisions about disability retirement or other life changes, should that become necessary.

2. The trip to England and France provided further insights into activities or situations that brought on symptoms—in this case, heat and crowds of people or events with a great deal of movement all around me. This was the first time I really understood that I needed to avoid crowded events and that I needed to stay as cool as possible, drinking water constantly on hot days. Vacations were useful opportunities to identify challenging activities because I was out of my normal routine and more able to devote energy to observation. Many vestibular patients have difficulty with crowd motion as well as heat.

3. Applying for a disability retirement was one of the most difficult decisions of my life. First, it was a very emotional decision because it was bound up so closely with my definition of who I was. It felt

like defeat, like failure. It also felt like I was giving up a huge part of my life. I couldn't imagine what it would be like to stop being a professional person. I was losing a big chunk of my identity and walking into the unknown with a chronic illness. There was also that nagging concern about not really being sick, which translated into not really deserving a disability. On the practical side, I was fortunate that my employer offered a disability based on my inability to perform my current job; that made the determination easier. I was required to file for Social Security disability, which focused on my ability to perform any useful work rather than my ability to do my current job. The Social Security application was denied, and I didn't have the energy to appeal. I understood this denial was a typical response, and even though it didn't affect my disability benefits it contributed to my feelings of failure, of being an undeserving failure. The decision to file for disability is a very difficult personal decision. If you must make this decision, seek out friends who have made the decision, professionals at your workplace and other resources to help you through the process.

6

A Clear Diagnosis at Last

NOVEMBER 1997–DECEMBER 1997

When I left work I did not make a miraculous recovery. During the first few weeks I felt a little sicker each day—nausea, headaches, aching muscles and joints, and numbing fatigue. When I was working I'd willed myself to keep going and ignore the symptoms. Now it was as if I'd slowly released my tight grip on the controls and the symptoms steadily increased.

November 4, 1997

After several weeks at home, it is finally clear to me that I am really sick. While it is not completely debilitating, I have only two to three hours of activity I am capable of each day. So far I am spending most of that time on walking or gardening . . . It feels great to have time alone again. It is great to have no pressure to go in a certain direction, no deadline for a decision about what is next. I feel that very deeply because I am in a small boat that has still not moved a great distance from the old harbor, it is clearly in view. I need patience.

November 7, 1997

I am into sort of a schedule where I rest almost all afternoon. Meaning I meditate for 30 to 45 minutes, I read, I sit and stare at the birds, I do my yoga. I actually can't admit to seeing any huge difference day to day. But I do see a difference from the exhaustion I felt working. I am much more in touch with my energy level. I can sense when I am getting tired and stop. So for the first time I am capable of doing what Dr. Loveless said: Keep up a certain level of activity but don't get tired. That never made sense before, I was always tired.

I was surprised to find I didn't miss work. My new job was healing. It was a relief not to make the Herculean effort required to succeed in a very difficult job; however, I did not understand the magnitude of the transition ahead. It was enough to be able to sleep late, to do a few simple chores, to take naps and read. It had been a very long time since I had experienced the luxury of time to rest and reflect.

I saw the months just after my retirement as a period of transition, a time dedicated to healing. It was important to have the patience to slow down and conserve my energy, to avoid becoming goal oriented and to keep my expectations realistic.

Fortunately, the six-month waiting period before my next round of vestibular testing with Dr. Black was now almost over. I felt a new sense of determination and clarity when I scheduled an appointment to resume the tests. The tough decision to make health my top priority had been made. My retirement and my commitment to focus time, energy, and attention on getting well was an important signal to Dr. Black. My commitment increased his commitment. He again explained that I exhibited symptoms of several different balance problems. Many balance problems have similar symptoms, but the treatment approaches are quite different. He needed to determine which specific condition affected me the most before recommending a treatment plan. He asked for several new tests, and he ordered the results from my past magnetic resonance imaging scan as well as the lumbar puncture.

Many balance problems have similar symptoms but the treatment approaches are quite different. Physicians need to determine which specific condition affects a person the most before recommending a treatment plan.

During November and early December I repeated the balance-related tests. I also started to write about my activity level, energy level, and general observations much more frequently.

November 16, 1997

It struck me Friday night, or early Saturday morning, 4:30 a.m., couldn't sleep, that I am open to getting well—really for the first time.

I did not realize that I spent so much energy just getting through my life, forcing myself to do what I needed, so I had no energy and no focus for getting well. It was a nice idea to contemplate after 4 weeks off work.

November 19, 1997

I had a very busy day today in a week I have been really taking it easy. I drank coffee at lunch. The caffeine was quite a stimulant! I saw real clearly how sometimes I feel if I just keep moving I can stay ahead of the wave of tiredness. But it began to creep in—like a fog over water—by 3:30 p.m.

I went back to confer with Dr. Black at the conclusion of the new round of testing in mid-December. His diagnosis was that my symptoms were caused by *perilymph fistulas*, rips or tears in a membrane in my inner ear. *Fistulas* are generally due to whiplash from car accidents, head trauma, or taking an airplane flight with blocked Eustachian tubes. He was puzzled because there had been no such triggering event in my case. I explained that, in fact, I did fly twice with a bad cold right before the problem started. All this time my records indicated the condition stemmed from a virus. I never realized it made any difference there was a flight involved.

> *Fistulas* are generally due to whiplash from car accidents, head trauma, or taking an airplane flight with blocked Eustachian tubes.

This new information increased Dr. Black's confidence in his diagnosis of rips in the inner ear membrane. I wondered whether my diagnosis and treatment would have been faster if I'd described the airplane flight in my initial appointments, but there was no value in dwelling on what was past.

Dr. Black also explained that my test results indicated fistulas in both ears as well as a condition called *endolymphatic hydrops*, secondary to the fistulas. Hydrops was basically a swelling inside the inner ear that caused many similar symptoms, but it was essential to treat the fistulas first. The treatment started with six to eight weeks of bed rest—carefully restricting pressure to the head, chest, or abdomen. Too much pressure—from sneezing, blowing one's nose, or even opening a jar—could reopen the fistulas. The bed rest is comparable to a cast on a broken limb; parts of the ear needed to be immobilized in order to heal. Dr. Black introduced me to his nurse, who described the procedures I would need to follow during this bed rest and provided a copy of the "fistula precautions." Both of them were delighted to have solved the mystery of what was wrong, of course, but no more delighted than I!

Endolymphatic hydrops is basically a swelling inside the inner ear that causes many symptoms similar to those caused by fistulas. The fistula treatment starts with bed rest—carefully restricting pressure to the head, chest, or abdomen. The bed rest is comparable to a cast on a broken limb; parts of the ear needed to be immobilized in order to heal.

I was so excited I failed to ask even basic questions like "Will I get well?" and "When should I start to feel better?" I even had to search the Internet for more information about perilymph fistulas when I got home. I had a diagnosis! I didn't know quite what it meant yet, but I had waited so long to know what was wrong that, for now, a diagnosis was enough.

$$* \quad * \quad *$$

Dr. Black's diagnosis ended a very confusing and frustrating two-year period. I hadn't been worried or fearful that I had a serious, life-threatening disease. My major emotional reaction, when I experienced any emotional reaction at all, was the sense of being powerless and not in control. During my twenty-five-year career I had developed an arsenal of skills to maintain control and power. Those skills were instrumental in both my career and many other parts of my life. They had largely failed me in managing this illness—so far.

In my work life I had no trouble calling in experts when I realized I didn't have the proper training or expertise to address a problem. Why was it so hard for me to accept help regarding this illness? I had welcomed the suggestions of friends and colleagues about treatments, nutrition, and practitioners, but these suggestions represented data gathering and problem solving. The hard-to-accept help involved assistance in living my life, in getting my share done. Taking disability retirement was the best example: I did not want to picture myself as someone who was forced to stop working because she was sick, as someone who could no longer make a contribution to the world of work. On a smaller scale, I still insisted on carrying heavy grocery bags up the thirty steps to the front door and doing the yard work.

As a well person, I'd made some rigid assumptions about what it meant to be sick: It was totally debilitating, it was dramatic and tragic, and it was fundamentally life limiting and life altering. These assumptions were now contradicted by my own experience. The events of my life as a sick person were identical to the events of my life as a well person. I still visited with friends, although now I tried to see only one at a time. I still went to the grocery store, although now I tried to limit myself to disciplined thirty-minute list-in-hand run-throughs. I still cleaned the house, although the chores I used to do in a few straight hours on one day I now spread out over three days. I still took vacations, and I still visited my family. I continued to do many of the same things I'd always done, perhaps fewer things, or for a shorter duration, but the basic ingredients of life were the same. Life is not completely full for healthy people and completely empty for sick people—there are shades of difference but not sharp outlines. This sameness and general lack of drama contributed to my continuing doubts about whether I was really sick.

This range of emotions passed like clouds across the landscape of my thoughts. In truth, few feelings penetrated the flatness. The flatness was a blessing, a form of self-protection. Aside from my crying jags, I was generally removed from all these feelings. They floated above and around me, but I did not spend a great deal of time or energy worrying about them. Flatness was not limited to my emotions about the illness. Most of the time I felt I was in a thick fog or like there was some sort of shield around me preventing direct contact with other people or even myself. Every once in awhile I perceived something significant, but it would generally slip away before I was able to respond. Things happened around me, but I rarely felt like a participant. It took most of my energy just to get through the day and to keep pushing for a diagnosis. Later, after the fog began to dissipate, I learned that *emotional flatness* is a particular symptom of vestibular illness.

＊　　＊　　＊

Throughout my illness one of the few emotions that consistently broke through the flatness was concern about my father. As I searched for a diagnosis, he was slowly succumbing to Alzheimer's disease. In the fall of 1996, a year before my retirement, he was also diagnosed with bladder cancer. My sisters, my stepmother, and I agreed it would be disastrous for him to go through chemotherapy or radiation treatments. Medications and hospitalization severely disoriented him, and his doctors did not feel these treatments were promising enough to warrant the side effects. The diagnosis of bladder cancer seemed like a mixed blessing because the alternative was an inexorable decline with Alzheimer's.

Dad's doctor said it was unlikely he would live more than six months after the cancer diagnosis. In 1997, after my retirement but before the diagnosis, Shelly and I went to North Carolina for Thanksgiving. Dad was still well enough for a family gathering: Dad, my stepmother, my mother, me and all my sisters, and all the grandchildren were there. Dad was in his element! Somehow he managed to recognize everyone, even my mother's cousin whom he had not seen in at least five years. He was so completely himself, laughing and telling stories, it was easy to forget he was sick at all. He was resting on a plateau and holding his own. He was doing so well that the threat of the cancer receded from the front of my mind.

Two weeks after I got home to Portland, right after Dr. Black ended the long search for a diagnosis, my youngest sister, Lynn, called. Dad was starting to experience some pain, and the doctors were having difficulty identifying the best pain medication. We knew that once pain medication started we would lose Dad. Our highest priority was that he should not suffer, but with the pain medication we knew he would become disoriented. The doctor told us this was the final stage of the cancer and that Dad would not live more than a few weeks. He deteriorated rapidly over the next week: The pain became worse, and the medication made Dad lose consciousness. I knew I wanted to be with him at the end. I put off my bed rest treatment. Shelly and I flew to North Carolina on December 23.

My father died on December 27. I was fortunate to be by his side with Shelly and my sister Anne. The funeral was two days later. We were all buoyed by the many former football players, coaches, and friends from different phases of Dad's life who attended the funeral. Each one came with new stories of good things Dad did for them, stories he'd never told. I went to North Carolina knowing I wanted to deliver the eulogy at his funeral. Without someone telling stories and making people laugh, as Dad would have, it would not be *his* funeral. As I got some of my biggest laughs, I could feel him there, smiling over my shoulder. For a few brief moments I was still his little girl, doing him proud.

That week was a dramatic example of running on adrenaline; it was simply more important to be fully immersed in the experience. This was the only time I was going to lose my father. I was afraid of his death, of the death of anyone close to me. I wanted not to shy away from the experience but to move into it, fully. More than anything I wanted to be at my father's side, to experience the closeness of my sisters and to be comforted by the rituals surrounding the funeral. I ignored my illness during the week I spent in North Carolina. In many ways it was a break from being sick.

By the time we drove to Raleigh to fly home to Portland, however, my adrenaline was gone. I collapsed. On the long flight I alternately slept, cried, and began to plan my six to eight weeks of bed rest. It was the middle of winter, gray and cold. I was sick. I was tired. I was so sad. The prospect of spending weeks in hibernation was a great comfort, and it matched my energy level perfectly.

Speaking From Experience: Tips to Make Your Journey Easier

1. When I retired on disability, all I saw were the losses, the downsides. Ever so slowly, I started to perceive the fundamental shift in my life from taking care of work to taking care of myself. I saw it as a choice to stop work, but it was actually a choice to put my health first. Once the choice was made, I began to understand that my new job was to get well, to take all the right steps to get my health back. This choice affected my attitude and dedication; it was also a clear signal to my doctors that I was serious about receiving and following their medical advice.

2. When Dr. Black presented me with a diagnosis of my vestibular problems, I was overwhelmed with emotion, almost disbelief. I was also alone and unprepared, which meant I failed to ask basic questions that caused me confusion throughout the early stages of my bed rest. Even though I knew better and had learned how valuable it was to have Shelly with me, I forgot to bring him at the critical moment. Any meeting with a doctor is a potential diagnosis and proposed treatment plan, so be sure to take someone with you, to take notes and ask questions. If you forget, it might make sense to schedule another appointment to clarify your questions.

3. I came home from my appointment and searched the Internet for information on perilymph fistulas. Thankfully, there is now a wealth of information about most vestibular disorders on the Internet. One particularly useful Web site is sponsored by the national Vestibular Disorders Association (www.vestibular.org).

7

Perilymph Fistulas—Bed Rest

JANUARY 1998–FEBRUARY 1998

B ed rest began January 7, 1998. Dr. Black gave me a short handout with a list of things I could not do—almost everything. I was allowed to be up, vertical, for ninety minutes a day, total. During my hour and a half I took a shower, went to the bathroom, and walked to the kitchen for food. The rest of the day I was confined to bed or a couch, with my head elevated all the time. I even had to sleep sort of sitting up, with my head elevated on a foam wedge. Shelly was working hard and traveling frequently. I couldn't cook or clean, grocery shop, or walk the dog. I could not just press on and do what needed to be done. The time limit was absolute. I had to get help.

Fortunately, I was able to hire a woman to grocery shop, do laundry, and cook, once a week. She had worked as a nanny and housekeeper for some good friends and was used to cooking healthy vegetarian dishes. She came every Monday and prepared several salads and casseroles to last through the week. She covered them with plastic wrap so I wouldn't have to struggle or exert any pressure on my ears to open tight-fitting lids. The microwave became a necessity to minimize standing up at the stove. I also hired my young neighbor Molly to come in once a day and walk Bunkee and collect the mail and the newspaper on the way up the steps. Being dependent on others and having my home life invaded by strangers felt very strange and uncomfortable, but there was no other choice.

My home is three stories high, and our bedroom is all the way up on the top floor. One of the instructions for bed rest was to minimize the use of stairs. I quickly got into a routine of getting up, showering, getting dressed,

57

and going downstairs for the day. This used up almost half my daily quotient of "vertical" time. Something about this morning ritual provided energy and order; it got me ready for my job—resting. The sunroom we had added the year before became my haven. There were windows on three walls and multiple skylights. It had the most light of any room in the house. Light was important for keeping my spirits up. Luckily it was also furnished with a recliner that became command central for the duration of the bed rest. Equipped with remote controls for the TV and the stereo, surrounded by books, and with a clear line of sight to the front door, there was little need to get up for interruptions.

I was exhausted from the recent North Carolina trip and the grief and other emotions surrounding my father's death. The first week went by in a blur. I took little naps all day long, meditated, read, and wrote down the thoughts and feelings floating by. I'd been cautioned not to get tired, to limit phone calls and visitors to avoid fatigue. I was careful and diligent about the bed rest guidelines. I did not want to have to do this again! The first week was very solitary; it took time to get used to how I felt, what I could do, what I needed help with, and preparing for the weeks ahead. I did not set foot outside the house for seven weeks.

January 13, 1998

Over the past week the grief has taken on a new pattern. It is not all consuming, the focus of my life. It is a powerful force that is triggered sometimes out of nowhere but always by small kindnesses.

There are other times like last night going to sleep when memories come to me strongly. Last night I was lightly thinking about the funeral and the eulogy. I recalled Dad's familiar "you don't know what you are talking about . . ." line and then, like before, actually felt Dad at my elbow. With his sideways grin and twinkle in his eye as he gave me that slight poke in the ribs and asked "when did you get to be such a smart aleck?" He was there and I felt it so strongly that it hurt to leave the memory. The memory of him is so close and real—slipping out of it is a stark reminder that he is not really here, ever again.

I am grateful for the bed rest and the solitude. It is allowing me not to "stuff" anything. It is allowing me to work through to some closure—an ending—in my father's life. That did not come for me with his passing. I can see that now. I don't wish not to be sad, for the grief to pass quickly. I'm not ready for that—the grief and the memories are all I have. They make me feel close to Dad. Hopefully

other emotions will arise to maintain the closeness without the pain.
But I don't regret the pain, it is a mirror for the love.

These emotions were too raw to talk about except with myself.

Shelly picked up all the slack around the house: additional food shopping, taking care of Bunkee and Looey, and doing special things for me. When Shelly was home he was essentially waiting on me. I really needed him, his support, his affection, and his presence. I decided to take a vacation from feeling guilty about being a wet blanket on our social life. This bed rest was our investment in the long term.

Life settled into its new pattern. Molly came by every day to walk Bunkee and get the mail. At first we both hesitated to just chat. I didn't want to impose by taking more of her time, and she was concerned about tiring me. Soon, though, I began to look forward to her short visits, and periodically we'd have longer chats. Our talks were a rare opportunity for me to get to know a bright young woman at a very formative period in her life. Our conversations took me back to the time right after my college graduation, my sense of expectancy, of insecurity about measuring up and of determination. Molly was even more idealistic, very hard on herself and dedicated to living her life in a way that made a difference. Her anticipation energized me. She was interested in my life's experiences. It was a moment—a space of time—when we were both slowed down enough and open enough to listen and enjoy each other's company.

My friend Julie visited every Friday afternoon. Julie was my first friend when I'd moved to Portland twenty years earlier; she was my yoga teacher. We lived about two blocks apart but with our busy lives struggled to see each other. The time we now spent visiting in the sunroom was a balm for my spirits and renewed and deepened our friendship. Julie's commitment to sit with me for a few hours every Friday despite her very busy life became as healing for her as it was for me. These small visits were an important part of the evolving structure of my solitude.

*   *   *

Shelly designed forms on the computer so I could keep detailed records of my symptoms, including what I was doing when they started and when they occurred during the day. It was important to him to document any emerging trends. He's even more analytical than I am; this information helped him feel a bit more control. He had watched, largely from the sidelines, for almost two years and he was now delighted to have a specific treatment plan to follow.

I began to have headaches every few days. They started the second week of the bed rest. I was also periodically dizzy even if I was not moving at all. By the beginning of the third week of bed rest, the headache was constant and I was unable to control the pain with aspirin or Tylenol. I was also experiencing the *scotomas*, or visual migraines, I'd first had in the summer of 1996. This time they were accompanied by what I assumed was the migraine. The worst headache began on Day 14 of bed rest and persisted to Day 20. Shelly was out of town on a business trip for several days, and I was getting desperate. On the morning of Day 20 the headache was so bad I called my friend Paul to ask for help. I considered calling Dr. Black's office but decided against it. They couldn't fix this; they could only tell me what was happening. I didn't care what was happening—I just wanted to fix it! Paul made an immediate house call.

By the time he arrived the pain in my head was so severe I was nauseated. It was a blessing to have a close friend who was a chiropractor and a healer. He asked me a few pertinent questions and began massaging my feet to reduce the nausea. Within minutes the nausea subsided, and he started to work on my headache by massaging my neck, head, and shoulders. He was very cautious because of the restrictions about any pressure on my head, chest, or abdomen and decided not to do any chiropractic adjustment. After just half an hour the headache was gone. As Paul talked to me calmly and massaged the horrible headache away, I started to cry: tears of relief, tears of gratitude.

Paul visited regularly after this acute episode. He had provided good counsel while I searched for a diagnosis. Now he was able to provide treatments that made the bed rest tolerable. I could not identify the cause of the headaches. They could be from sitting all day and holding my head and spine in awkward positions or part of the fistulas healing. Either way, headaches were the worst part—physically—of the bed rest.

In Week 4 I was hit with unending dizziness. The dizziness was worse in certain positions—when I turned my head to the right or leaned even slightly—and it never abated. After a few days, I called Dr. Black's office and spoke to the nurse. She thought this sounded like a hydrops "episode." She recommended I eat and drink carefully over the day to balance my intake and to avoid too much salt or sugar. Normally, the inner ear structure maintains constant fluid levels independent of the body. After an injury the fluid levels in the ear can fluctuate with changes in overall body fluids. The objective of the hydrops diet was to maintain constant fluid levels in the body so that fluid levels in the ear did not vary substantially. I was probably not drinking enough fluids. I added what and when I ate and drank to the list of things I was recording.

> Normally, the inner ear structure maintains constant fluid
> levels independent of the body. After an injury the fluid levels
> in the ear can fluctuate with changes in overall body fluids.

When Dr. Black explained my diagnosis back in December 1997, he told me I had perilymph fistulas as well as hydrops in both ears. He showed me diagrams of the structures in the inner ear and explained each condition. He explained the need to treat the fistulas first: That was the bed rest. That was the part I remembered most clearly. The hydrops diet was a part of the handout package his nurse provided. I hadn't realized that I would need to "multi-task": do bed rest *and* deal with hydrops. I had no clue about how to distinguish dizziness due to hydrops from dizziness due to fistulas. This hydrops episode was the beginning of my education about many different types of dizziness, their causes, and their treatments. Trying to sort out which dizziness was which would take years. Developing a vocabulary to describe all the permutations of "dizzy" would take even more time.

Between the hydrops and the headaches, the last few weeks of bed rest were like following a delicate soufflé recipe you are trying for the first time: Constant vigilance was required. At the first sign of dizziness or a headache, I whipped out one of my three defenses. Sometimes it was simple, like an ordinary headache remedy: I had to be careful to avoid headache remedies with caffeine. They were dehydrating and weren't good for the hydrops. Paul came every other day to give me a massage. He also brought over some of his medical books with drawings of the internal parts of the ear. Studying those illustrations helped me understand both conceptually and visually what was going on inside my body. Sticking with the hydrops diet was a constant. The diet, the headache remedies, the massages, and the knowledge all contributed some small semblance of order and control and reduced my sense of being a powerless victim.

After five weeks of bed rest I was anxious and depressed: anxious that I was seeing no progress and depressed that the bed rest was not working.

February 11, 1998

I am about 5 weeks into 7 weeks of bed rest. These last few days have been ones of emotional crisis. Today, and often yesterday, I felt myself on the verge of tears. I feel confused—about how to help myself spiritually, about the source of my pain (the healing or the mourning), and maybe about how to control this. As I write this somewhere I know that I am in God's hands—that the healing and the grieving will resolve as they should when they should—and I still feel a need not to be passive. To contribute the peace and positive energy of my meditations, to pray those thoughts are consistent with truth and to be grateful for the many miracles around me—which I have slowed down enough to see.

In the midst of this crisis of confidence I realized I hadn't really asked much about what I would feel during the bed rest. I needed some reassurance from Dr. Black. I called his nurse, who told me some patients did feel a difference when the fistulas closed.

Patients often can actually pinpoint a specific time when their perceptions and balance changed. Other patients gradually get better but did not perceive a single point of dramatic change. The nurse also told me that my next appointment would be just fifteen minutes, a quick progress check. The only way to know whether the fistulas were healed was to increase my activity and record the symptoms over the next six months.

Six months! My hope for a rapid cure seemed dashed again. I had completely forgotten the longer term aspects of the treatment regime. After that initial "Oh no!" I realized it was reassuring to hear there was still a possibility the bed rest was successful. It was also valuable to be reminded (again!) not to look for dramatic or conclusive developments at my next appointment.

This was familiar territory: the cycle of frustration–action–hope–despair. I'd expected to feel different when the fistulas closed. Because there was no "A-ha!" moment when I suddenly felt better, I thought the fistulas were not closed. After days of reflection I realized that I still expected an instant cure, that one day I would wake up and be well, that this illness would be over and all this would be behind me. Here was my first inkling that perhaps the treatment would be like the diagnosis: a slow and painstaking process, with two steps forward and one step back.

Several days before my quick fifteen-minute progress check appointment with Dr. Black, I reviewed my notes. As I looked back over the full seven-week period I could see that the bouts of dizziness were decreasing. When I started on bed rest I was constantly dizzy, whether I was sitting still or moving. In recent weeks, since I'd changed how I ate and drank to deal with the hydrops, only certain movements or positions seemed to make me dizzy. On the other hand, some of the most dramatic incidents or spikes in dizziness had occurred recently, in the evenings. I was recording less pressure in my ears, especially in the past two weeks. The changes were subtle, and I was not confident they represented a trend, but my notes confirmed my perceptions. There was no change in my ears ringing; they both rang constantly and loudly. I also still had the periodic headaches. The most noticeable positive changes were in my energy level and my appetite. I didn't know what any of this meant, or whether it was important, but it felt good to step back and look at the overall picture and see some bits of what seemed to be progress.

There was no question whether Shelly would go with me to this appointment. This was my first foray outside the house in seven weeks! I was thrilled to just go down the front steps and get in the car; it felt like I was emerging from a cocoon. I had no stamina; the slightest exertion left me weak and shaky. It was a challenge to walk from the car into the medical office. This was more interesting than disappointing; I wasn't concerned about rebuilding my physical conditioning. That was something to look forward to.

Dr. Black's office is on the third floor of the medical building. Should I take the stairs or risk the quick pressure buildup of an elevator ride? I was too weak to risk the stairs, so we got in the elevator and pressed the button for the second floor, got out, and rested to let my ear pressure acclimate. Once we finally arrived at the third floor Dr. Black's staff was waiting to take me into the treatment room immediately. They knew this first post-bed rest appointment was a huge physical challenge.

When I handed Dr. Black my typed summary of weekly progress, and a sample of the daily symptom tracking form, he broke into a huge grin. This was a double confirmation: First, I was engaged and energetic enough to prepare this summary, which meant I was recovering, and second, the symptom tracking data themselves showed that I was recovering.

Dr. Black thought the headaches could be related to the fistulas because of pressure change or fluid leakage in my ears. He thought chiropractic adjustments to relieve the headaches were acceptable if they did not put pressure on the fistulas.

Dr. Black explained that some of my other symptom patterns indicated hydrops. The symptoms for fistula and hydrops were quite similar, but they had different causes. The fistula symptoms came with exertion or pressure. The more constant hydrops symptoms were caused by diet and fluids or even weather changes. It was hard for me to understand this at first. It was like learning a new language. It took me a long while to get fluent. I tried to use this new understanding for tracking what caused the headaches and then adjusting my diet before the hydrops progressed for several days.

Dr. Black was pleased with the progress I described and emphasized that the next six weeks were as important to the healing as the complete bed rest had been. He advised me to s-l-o-w-l-y increase daily activity, building up to four to six hours by the end of the six-week period. I had to avoid pressure on my head, chest, or abdomen, but at least I could stand up and walk around! The rest of the time I was to stay in bed or recline. If I experienced any dizziness or ear pressure, I was to stop the activity immediately and remain still, starting up again only when the symptoms were gone. Dr. Black referred to this approach as "sneaking up" on activity. He emphasized that my usual mode of "pushing through" was unacceptable. Even if the fistulas were closed, the connective tissue was not yet healed. Full recovery—complete healing of the fistulas—was going to take a year.

We asked about next steps. What if the bed rest and incremental activity were not successful? Dr. Black described a surgical procedure available to repair the fistulas but said he thought the associated risks to my hearing and the possibility of exacerbating other conditions, such as hydrops, meant surgery wasn't a good choice. Because I had fistulas in both ears, I was looking at a year for surgery and full recovery for each ear because he did not recommend performing surgery on both ears at once.

Both Shelly and I were grateful for Dr. Black's expertise and for his recommendation of a treatment largely based on letting the body heal itself. Despite my earlier doubts about whether I could see improvement, Dr. Black's explanations reassured us.

February 25, 1998

I completed the 7 weeks of bed rest and went to see Dr. Black yesterday. He is optimistic, although I was clear that I see subtle changes (meaning I don't have confidence in them) in level and frequency of dizziness and ear pressure. I see no changes in tinnitus [ringing in the ears]. But I am certain that my personal energy and appetite are better. I can build slowly to 4–6 hours "up" a day, lifting more, sleeping lower. I was totally exhausted after the office

visit—tearful even. I feel cautiously optimistic . . . and I was so "down"
because I didn't think it had worked. Now we'll see—if the symptoms
come back, it didn't work.

In many ways, the preparation for this appointment was a sign I was
getting better. The ability to record symptoms and perceive a pattern and
have that confirmed by the doctor boosted my confidence in the diagnosis
as well as the treatment. At the very least I had succeeded in getting my
activity level below my energy level for six weeks.

This was good news, considering that the only way to further decrease
my activity level was to go into a coma!

Speaking From Experience: Tips to Make Your Journey Easier

1. Bed rest marked my first awareness of the distinction between fistula-
   related dizziness and hydrops-related dizziness. The dizziness was
   constantly recurring, so it was necessary to track back whenever I was
   dizzy to try to find the cause. Had I just sneezed? Lifted something?
   Pulled open the refrigerator door? If so, that was exertion, and the
   dizziness might be due to an open fistula. If I couldn't find a cause, or
   if the dizziness was more constant, it was more likely to be hydrops
   related. The more astute I became at identifying the root causes, the
   trigger activities, the better my treatment would be. This was concrete
   validation for active participation in my recovery and accurate symptom
   tracking.

2. Tracking symptoms during bed rest became my full-time focus.
   After about a week I was able to develop a checklist of symptoms—
   dizziness, nausea, headache, ear ringing, vertigo—that I monitored
   throughout the day. I noted when they occurred as well as how severe
   the symptoms were. To make this easier, I typed up a table on the
   computer so I had a record to fill in for each day. I also left space for
   any new or unusual symptoms and a space to jot notes or questions.
   Before I went to my seven-week check with Dr. Black I summarized the
   trends I saw from my notes and typed it up to present to him. I didn't
   feel confident that my observations were reliable, but they were a start,
   better than nothing. I ended my career to focus on my health, so this
   was my work. You are the only person who can identify how you are
   feeling. If you don't track your symptoms and progress, then all the
   doctor has to go on is one face-to-face appointment every seven weeks.

3. The questions I failed to ask Dr. Black when he diagnosed my vestibular illness in December plagued me through the first stage of bed rest and were finally answered at the first post-bed rest checkup. In December, I failed to comprehend the long time period for all the stages of the bed rest. I also assumed there was some magical test that would tell me whether or not the bed rest had worked to heal the fistula. At the seven-week checkup I faced two realities. First, there was still a great deal of uncertainty about the pace and direction of my treatment; those depended on my body's response at each stage. Also, this treatment was going to take a long time—measured in months and years rather than days or weeks.

8

Perilymph Fistulas—
Neighborhood Rest

MARCH 1998–MAY 1998

The day after my appointment with Dr. Black, in my excitement at more "up time," I did too much and put myself right back in bed for a few days. I decided then and there to get myself on a disciplined schedule. It was simply too tempting to go hog wild strolling around the block, sorting laundry, and paying bills after two months of inactivity!

Therefore, every morning I put together a daily schedule and stuck to it. I had seven weeks to work up to four to six hours of activity a day, so I figured I could increase my daily "up" time thirty to forty-five minutes each week. A half hour did not sound like very much, but it was free time, not time I had to spend in the shower, the bathroom, or making meals. Even those few more "up" minutes included delicious new freedoms. I was able to sit at the desk or the computer. I could use the stove again! I could take short car rides on flat roads, and I could begin to go outside in the yard. On the other hand, I still couldn't lift anything more than five pounds (you'd be amazed at how many things weigh more than five pounds!). There could be no bending down or putting my head below my heart (. . . and no sex!). I couldn't go up to high altitudes—such as 500 feet. The restriction on altitude was particularly interesting because I lived in Portland's West Hills neighborhood, already at a higher elevation than the central city and one filled with sudden steep inclines.

After a few days of rest I started twice-daily forays into the great outdoors. The first day it was only out to get the newspaper and a short fifty-yard walk to the street corner. In the afternoon I walked around the yard, a pretty short trip given it was a 5,000-square-foot lot, but it felt like a big step forward. Every day, I tried to walk a little farther in my slow, cautious way. The only one more excited about this was my dog, Bunkee. Even though she continued her daily walks with Molly the dog walker, these small trips around the street were her job. She was busy again!

These walks were central elements of my healing. They allowed me to get outdoors, test my balance with a fairly routine activity, and observe the results. These walks provided the clearest measure—immediately and over the coming months—of my remaining problems and progress.

At the end of two weeks I could walk about a quarter mile and climb the first hill near our house, which had about a fifty-foot rise in elevation. It took me another two weeks to build up to strolling half a mile.

During the uphill parts of the walk I paid close attention to the pressure in my ears. If the pressure did not clear when I paused for a few moments, that was the signal I needed to turn around and descend. I became expert at detecting slight changes in ear pressure and discerning whether the pressure cleared. The ability to perceive these changes seemed mysterious and incomprehensible when Dr. Black first mentioned it, but it quickly became natural and easy.

I'd also discovered during my walks that when I turned my head to the side or shifted my focus while I was walking, I drifted to one side—my feet followed my eyes or my head. This phenomenon is one type of ataxia and is a common symptom of balance problems.

Just when I was getting the hang of detecting changes in ear pressure I had another major episode of dizziness and nausea. Dr. Black had described the difference between symptoms from fistula (related to exertion) and those from hydrops (symptoms are "out of the blue," fluctuating independent of activity or movement), but it took me several days to realize the dizziness and nausea were due to hydrops and respond by changing my diet and fluids. I was still learning and not yet expert at distinguishing the difference. It would be years before I had confidence identifying a hydrops episode. Although it sounded simple, elusive complications such as barometric pressure changes, or even temperature fluctuations from other infectious processes, could, in addition to diet, trigger hydrops episodes. Figuring out what caused the hydrops was hard enough. Distinguishing dizziness and imbalance due to hydrops from episodes due to fistulas was difficult even for a vestibular specialist.

This hydrops episode was a sharp reminder of the illness, and it snapped me backward both emotionally and physically for more than a week. These episodes were also a signal that the cycle of frustration–action–hope–despair was going to be with me for awhile. As long as I could observe some progress I remained hopeful. When some new symptoms or old symptoms reemerged it damaged my confidence, my hope. At least now I knew what action to take—modify my diet—and it worked fairly reliably, but when I was in the middle of an out-of-control hydrops episode I lost my hopeful perspective.

March 1998

There are some very important things I am learning and relearning. The first is about letting go. There have been many times during this illness when I had to have the discipline to do what I needed to do—whether it was doctors, medication, rest, nutrition, whatever—and then the ability or insight to let go. And realize there is a part of this that I can't control. Over the past two months that has recurred with a vengeance. I sat or reclined for 7 weeks. It was sometimes or mostly fine because I am a determined person. But at 5–6 weeks, when I did not think it had worked, I lost hope and got depressed. Somewhere in those depths, I saw that the rest was God's part; that I needed God's help and that it would come when it came. So for awhile I have let go. Sometimes I am troubled that I have a pattern of strong determination, disillusionment and depression and then I can let go, only then. But maybe it is like anything else; once I learn it I will move through those stages more effortlessly. I am grateful that I see the pattern so clearly and that I can let go.

This slow progress continued throughout March and the first week of April. I was still neighborhood bound, if not housebound, but I was able to do more and more. Almost every new activity caused an increase in dizziness, nausea, or headaches for awhile, but if I was diligent about "sneaking up" the symptoms declined slowly over time.

One of the ways to get beyond the neighborhood was weekend car rides. They became our major social outing. Shelly and I were limited to the flat parts of Portland, so we explored sections of the city we could not recall visiting in years. Unfortunately as we tried to extend their length I got nauseated from riding in the car, so this new avenue of amusement had to be curtailed.

Throughout these weeks after bed rest I kept notes on how I felt. At first the symptom charts were packed with bouts of dizziness, nausea, and all the other symptoms, along with what I'd been doing when the symptoms started. Those incidents decreased to only one or two a day if I sat in my command post chair in the sunroom, but now I was testing limits and regrouping; I was "sneaking up" on different activities.

I made steady progress, but it was not straightforward. Several good days were followed by setbacks that sent me back to command central in the sunroom. It was frustrating. I had to work hard for patience to let the healing move at its own pace. I began to understand that recovery from the fistulas was going to be a meditation on patience.

March 30, 1998

Almost at the end of my first stage after total bed rest. I have definitely felt better but it is slower than I ever imagined. I am walking almost a mile a day—largely on the flat part of the main neighborhood street. If I try to climb the cross street above it I feel a great deal of ear pressure so I'll "sneak up" on it. I have symptoms—dizziness, ataxia, lightheadedness—when I walk, garden, vacuum. The drama of hydrops has recurred once and I am still getting nauseous riding in the car. I feel I am getting well—even though it is very slow and I get discouraged at times. There is a new strength and a new personal energy.

✳   ✳   ✳

I was confident I was feeling better, and for my next appointment with Dr. Black I was prepared with the long list of symptoms, most notably the nausea from riding in a car and the recurrent hydrops. It was more and more rewarding to keep track of symptoms because I was learning which symptoms were relevant. I brought a lengthy progress report with me to the appointment.

Dr. Black decided I was ready to move to the next stage. Like before, this new stage meant small additions to everyday activity. Again, he was careful to emphasize that I should view all activity as an experiment. I needed to avoid inflexible commitments and responsibilities. It was important to continue observing symptoms closely and stop immediately when symptoms flared up. He thought the nausea in the car should go away as I began to drive—driving was allowed in this next stage! (I hadn't been this thrilled about driving since I got my first license!) There were still restrictions on the amount of lifting I could do, and I was not allowed to go above 800 feet elevation.

Swimming gently and only on the surface, walking, and using an exercise bike with no resistance were all on the approved list now. I was close to eighty percent healed, but I was cautioned to use great care with any head, chest, or abdominal pressure. I might always need to take care in bending down, even for simple things like tying my shoes. I accepted the cautions for now, but of course I was more hopeful for the future.

Dr. Black also mentioned that the hydrops generally resolved within the first year after fistulas close, but medications were available if it didn't.

Because my symptoms had decreased and my activity increased I was convinced the fistulas were closed. I placed too much importance on that particular milestone. It was necessary but not sufficient for my recovery. When I reread my notes from the December 1997 visit, the day I received a diagnosis, I noticed Dr. Black said the bed rest was *six to eight weeks in bed* plus *three months of very restricted activity.* I had remembered only the "six to eight weeks" part. I still clung to my idea of the immediate cure, even after two years of contrary experience. Most days I was satisfied with my progress, but periodically I was invited to an event, received an invitation from a friend to go to lunch, or simply tried to clean the house for too long and was confronted with the limits of a very narrow life.

April 24, 1998

I am gaining confidence I can feel good again . . . if not 100% then 90 or 95%. As I move back into activity the symptoms recede but it is very slow. Each new activity causes new symptoms and I have a constant vigil against hydrops. The nausea riding in the car appears to be subsiding based on my "training" drives behind the wheel. I am just finishing a full week of feeling good by being careful, resting between activities, and drinking constantly. I am both hopeful and grateful. It is especially gratifying to be enjoying sex again, to be able to walk in the park, to be able to work in the garden and not be totally housebound.

At the same time there are things I want to retain from my just past life. I would like to retain the time to be a good friend. I would like to continue to reflect and meditate—to be open to what is next. I'd like to continue to draw. . .

71

This stage is one in which I need to be very careful—both for my health and to establish some new patterns that feed my soul—that bring more meaning and joy into this life.

When I walked into his office for my appointment, Dr. Black said "Oh! How wonderful. We are starting to see your personality emerge." I had no idea what he meant.

During the next week I began to realize that the emotional flatness and the fog were lifting. The invisible shield between me and the rest of the world was disappearing. It was such an elusive symptom; I hadn't even realized it was all connected to the balance problem. The interest in new things and the energy I felt were signals of a return—to myself. It was spring, and I wanted to bounce back, to feel great—something I hadn't felt for more than two years.

✳   ✳   ✳

I couldn't fly for a year after bed rest because of the potential damage to my ears. Because I was earthbound, several family members decided to come visit me. The first visit was from Mom in May. Unlike some people, I did not feel any "must clean, must prepare" panic about Mom visiting. We just chatted, worked a large jigsaw puzzle, and teased each other about who was hiding the pieces—even though she clearly was the one misplacing all of them. I found her sitting on one! Actually, it turned out that Looey, the cat, was guilty of knocking loose pieces down and under the table when we took breaks. We had a very good time.

My mother knits beautifully. She has supplied daughters, sons-in-law, and grandchildren with sweaters for decades. We decided to purchase some yarn for a new sweater while she was in town. My normal yarn shop was closed, so we tried a new place. It was weird from the moment we entered the door. There were a few "Laurel and Hardy" incidents with the shop owner, but the real clincher came when I asked if she had any pale yellow, lightweight wool yarn. She replied "Yes, of course" with great enthusiasm and promptly brought us several skeins of bright salmon pink yarn. Mom and I burst out laughing. I giggled so uncontrollably we were forced to leave the store. I was not alone; my mother made a brief attempt at courtesy and then she doubled over with laughter as well. A color blind clerk in a yarn store?! I hadn't laughed so freely and totally in more than two years. The fog was lifting. I wasn't well, but I was better, and best of all I wasn't any worse.

Speaking From Experience: Tips to Make Your Journey Easier

1. The approach of "sneaking up" on activities was not only useful, it was required. If I had symptoms, I immediately stopped what I was doing and sat down. By repeating the same activity several times a day, or day after day, I could readily see if I was improving by noting how long it took for the symptoms to start. For example, I was able to walk just a little further and a little higher up the hill every day. This same repetition of activity also allowed me to recognize new symptoms—like ataxia while walking. My life was a laboratory where I observed symptoms and repeated activities to note any changes.

2. It was more rewarding to track symptoms as time went on because I was able to observe some progress. I presented the following information to Dr. Black in April 1998 so he could assess my progress during bed rest:

Conclusions for April 9, 1998:

BETTER:

- Fewer symptoms with low-level exertion: lifting, bending down, and going up and down stairs.
- Less ear pressure, dizziness and shakiness when walking. Can walk faster than at first. Walking up to a mile in the hills.
- Pulsing dizziness in the evenings is lessened.
- Ataxia when walking still occurs with head movement but less often.
- Less positional dizziness lying on right side.

SAME:

- Tinnitus is the same, ears ring constantly.
- Episodic headaches are still occurring and are difficult.

NEW (THESE SYMPTOMS CONFUSE MY SENSE OF WHAT I CAN DO):

- Riding in the car makes me nauseous every time. It is better with my eyes closed.
- Hydrops episodes—constant or pulsing dizziness—occur after car rides or when I don't observe the diet rigorously. Last episode March 15–March 20.
- Seem to have good days and bad days with no clear cause.

3. At this early stage of recovery I got my first inkling of what a long, slow process it was going to be. A few words—"meditation on patience"—spoke volumes. My past life had been primarily concerned with action. Certainly, there were moments and times of reflection, but the balance weighed heavily toward action. This was a new frontier where action needed to be held in close control and reflection was the leader. Like so many things I encountered and observed, this focus on the need for patience would emerge, fade away, and reemerge for years. If there is any lesson my vestibular disorder taught me, it was patience.

9

Hydrops Holding Me Back

JUNE 1998–AUGUST 1998

My next step in getting well was vestibular rehabilitation. I couldn't start that until the hydrops resolved. Vestibular therapy involved retraining my vision and muscles to work with (rather than against) my newly repaired ears so my balance system was functioning again. As long as I had the hydrops my ears were not a stable part of the system—they were sending the wrong balance signals to my brain—so any time spent in therapy would be wasted. Dr. Black explained that my experience was normal; hydrops frequently accompanies fistula closure and could be an issue for as long as a year.

> Hydrops frequently accompanies fistula closure and can be an issue for as long as a year.

My biggest fear was reopening the fistulas. Reopened fistulas meant back to square one with bed rest and months of recovery. During every hydrops episode I was unable to readily control, I worried first and foremost about fistulas because the symptoms were so similar. It seemed like every time I increased my activity or reduced my diligence, there was the hydrops.

I wasn't frustrated that I was unable to move immediately into the therapy. By now I was comfortable with the regimen and I understood I needed to persevere over the summer with patience and determination. I didn't have the same confidence in my ability to make progress with hydrops, but it was now clear that hydrops was a central concern.

I was also concerned that my stamina was not improving as steadily as I thought was necessary. I was able to do new activities as the weeks went by, but I was easily fatigued and felt tired and totally empty. I thought the chronic fatigue remained a complicating factor even if it was not the core problem. Dr. Loveless thought my energy should return about a year after I eliminated my balance problems and reduced my activity level below my energy level. I decided to take a proactive step to accelerate the time period.

I decided to try acupuncture. A good friend was seeing an acupuncturist who was helping her both with pain and with her energy level. I set up an appointment with Dr. Z. F. Lin, a practitioner of traditional Chinese medicine, including acupuncture. Because her father was an MD in China she was familiar with Western medicine and respectful of the contributions of both medical approaches. I gave her my medical history and described the diagnosis I had received as well as the treatment I was following. She listened respectfully and politely explained that her diagnosis was not based on the same principles and approaches. The symptoms she was interested in were basic functions, such as sleep, appetite, and bowel movements. She examined me and developed a treatment plan based on the finding of deficient kidney "chi." She recommended acupuncture treatments twice a week.

It was not long before these visits became an essential part of my life. Acupuncture was not a miracle cure; it worked very slowly. After a month or so I began to see small changes in my energy. At first I was extremely tired after each treatment but felt more energetic the next day. As the treatments progressed, my energy was markedly better immediately after the sessions and for the next few days. I also began to sleep more soundly. These early results were the main reason I continued treatments with Dr. Lin, but there were other reasons I was drawn to her as well.

Acupuncture is not a miracle cure; it works really slowly. But it helps.

Dr. Lin was a healer both with her needles and with her presence. She began every session by asking how I was doing. She gave me advice about diet; she told me I would not recover my energy with a vegetarian diet, that

I must eat fish for protein. She asked me about the pace of my life, whether I was resting enough, building a savings account of energy or spending it all. This was her version of keeping my activity below my energy level. As she administered the needles, she provided advice and told me anecdotes about her former patients. She offered endless encouragement and scolded me soundly when I needed it. Her wisdom about balance and its presence in all aspects of our bodies and our lives was exactly what I needed to hear. With the ups and downs of my healing process it was comforting to have someone to assess my progress regularly and suggest small corrections, someone knowledgeable to provide perspective.

June 18, 1998

There seem to be an endless stream of things that one could do to fill their life—all of which have the potential to be filled with meaning— but if I try stringing together too many in too short a time, it all ends up a jumble. Coming from my current place, it is hard to imagine how I got up and went to work for the past two years. It is all a blur at this point. I spoke to Joan in Dr. Black's office yesterday about my current downturn in health. She was reassuring that it didn't sound like reopened fistulas because the symptoms were not related to exertion. She reminded me that this would be slow with many ups and downs not a straight line with a strong upward slant. So now I see I have been doing too much, pushing progress—and I need to regroup. Deep inside I was not comfortable, not ready, but my old self thought I should be.

June 1998 was a month of new beginnings. I was now able to conduct "normal activity." I still had to pay attention: If I experienced any symptoms, I needed to back off and rest. I was leaving the cocoon of sickness and reemerging into the responsibilities and the pleasures of a whole life, but a whole life with limits. The bed rest and the limited activity had been a refuge; I was restricted in my normal activities but freed up to take care of myself and to think only of my healing. Although I'd experienced constant symptoms throughout the day—nausea, dizziness, vertigo, headache, muscle aches—I believed these symptoms would disappear as my body adapted to each new activity. As I now reentered the world, I saw things with fresh eyes and felt some very old pressures.

One of the first things I noticed was Shelly. He was overloaded both from his work and from supporting me. He worked all the time and traveled two to three weeks a month. He was leading a capital campaign at our synagogue, the first in thirty years. He was also doing everything around the house. I was now ready to resume a substantial part of the household management; it was better for both of us if I contributed more. It was natural to assume the responsibility for the household bills and the other business of running our home. I also started to search for elements of his business or the synagogue capital campaign where I could assist him.

At the same time I began to feel I should be working or doing something productive in addition to trying to get well. Some days I felt totally aimless and useless. There was no question it was too early, but I felt pressure to figure out what I was going to do now that I was getting well. This was completely self-imposed pressure, and it was counterproductive. The feeling of being useless and aimless recurred about every six weeks for the next year. I was grateful for the disability retirement annuity and the financial freedom it provided; it allowed me to feel I was contributing to the household without working. But the feelings of uselessness were a holdover from my past career; it said more about how I was accustomed to valuing myself. If I was unable to point to ongoing contributions, if I was devoid of pressing goals and demands, then I was not a productive person, a useful person.

In these early stages of recovery helping Shelly was the best way to channel and manage these emotions. It provided the flexibility I needed to consider all new activities as experiments and to back off and adjust the schedule when I was not feeling well.

June 22, 1998

Shelly is heading out of town until Wednesday. It feels fine, spacious in fact. It is more restful to have only my own pace to account for—but restful doesn't make for a whole life. So it is even better when Shelly is here, if a bit breakneck. I am so sympathetic with all the pressure that he must feel—all the deadlines and client demands. I hope to be able to help him get it more in balance. Dr. Lin has reminded me of that word . . . "balance." It is almost impossible to do without reflection, which is almost impossible without time.

I began by learning some new computer skills: how to use large spreadsheets to track pledges and donations for the synagogue's capital campaign. I also helped Shelly prepare a strategic plan for the capital campaign and worked with a graphic designer to produce a fund-raising brochure. I could work for about an hour, then I needed to rest. If the work involved meeting with other people, it exhausted me. I learned to view each event as an experiment and to slow down each time I got too involved. This pattern of overdoing and recuperating was difficult because it forced me to adjust my thinking, not just my activity. I had to learn that I didn't need to take as much responsibility as possible to be helpful. I could accommodate my abilities, do small things around the edges, and still contribute value.

At the same time I continued to reflect about the value of my career. I wasn't angry or disappointed, but I hadn't achieved any closure. It was still a nagging dilemma.

June 29, 1998

> *So this morning there was an article about BPA (Bonneville Power Administration) in the paper. Something like "prices look low and customers are rushing to sign up for power." I had a reaction that seemed important—because it caused me to rethink my sense of success and failure. I judged myself a failure despite my best efforts (sometimes more than I could sustain) at making it a better place to work and developing/implementing a strategy which could succeed. What the paper said is that the strategy could and did succeed. Although it sounds simple now there were times when it was far from clear. . . . For the first time today I can see I was too hard on myself. . . . When a person does their best and moves from their heart, the world is affected whether it is clear at that moment or not. All we can know is how we approached the task. So I will suspend my judgment of my own success or failure—I tried my best, I benefited from trying, I am honored to have had the chance, that is enough.*

I was reaching the final stage in the process of ending my career. The events that occurred at Bonneville Power Administration no longer affected me, and I was able to regain my sense of accomplishment and joy at a fulfilling career. My professional life was behind me.

＊　　＊　　＊

Meanwhile, my youngest sister, Lynn, and her family were coming to Oregon for a week in July. I was really looking forward to the visit and did some serious planning because I wanted to do as much as possible. The serious planning centered around what outings they would enjoy and what trips I could tolerate. The most absorbing part of the planning was trying to determine the precise altitude of the passes on the highway to the Oregon Coast. The coast was a perfect destination but there is a 3,000-foot mountain range—appropriately called the Coast Range—between Portland and the coast. I was only able to go up to about 1,200 to 1,500 feet in early July.

I purchased all the maps I could find and tried to determine the lowest pass over the mountains. The maps were not sufficiently precise, so I made phone calls and discovered that the information I was seeking—the precise altitude of various auto routes—was not readily available. Shelly called outdoor stores and bicycle shops, to see if bicyclers had a favored low-pass route, and then he focused in on the state highway department. He ended up getting the best information from the district employees who plowed snow from the road in the winter. Armed with their information we now knew 1,300 feet was the lowest pass. We picked several points in Portland with similar altitudes and took several training drives. This wasn't as quick and breezy as just hopping in the car and going off to the coast, but it was fun to investigate and find out about the altitudes. I would find this again and again: The new, slower, more deliberate way of doing things was not drudgery.

The night before Lynn and her family arrived I was able to ride all the way up the steep drive to Pittock Mansion, at 1,200 feet. This accomplishment relieved some of my anxiety about the drive to the coast. My fear was we'd all get about seventy-five miles from Portland and have to turn around because my ears would not clear. Turning around was fine for Shelly, but not fine for two kids looking forward to a beach trip. I was anxious not to spoil the enjoyment for everyone or upset their expectations. Plus, we'd made hotel reservations at the coast.

This was the first event or series of events that went beyond pure experiment. Up to this point I would sneak up on an event, and if it didn't appear to be working I just passed on it and backed down. But now I didn't feel that I could back down. This was real life!

We made the "high" altitude trip to the coast for the weekend a few days after Lynn and her family arrived. I was aware of significant pressure in my ears as we gained altitude and kept drinking water to clear my ears. I kept my eyes straight ahead because looking out the side window nauseated me. I was able to keep clearing the pressure from my ears, and once we were over the pass we stopped and celebrated. The celebration mostly involved finding a bathroom to deal with all the water I had been drinking! For the rest of the drive I couldn't help smiling from ear to ear and talking a blue streak. Driving to the coast had never been a big deal before, but this time it felt as momentous as climbing Mount Hood.

For the duration of their visit I pretended I was a normal person enjoying the summer. We went to a street fair in Portland. We went for a short hike in the Columbia River Gorge, my favorite loop with a trail leading under a waterfall and over a bridge crossing a steep chasm. It was such a pleasure to watch the kids explore.

July 6, 1998

Went to the rodeo yesterday in Molalla. It was a 50 mile drive each way and a more raucous event than I was used to. I felt pretty awful when I got home—muscle aches, nausea and sort of a rolling dizziness. I rested and slept for two hours and felt a lot better but still tired. Today I am still shaky and I notice my eyes doing some jumpy/flashy vision. The other side of the rodeo was that it felt good to be a normal person for a day. It was fun to be in a small rural community, to do something wholesome, just have an experience. So even though it was not that appealing to be sick, it was good to be alive.

July 13, 1998

Back to normal, sort of. Lynn, Rusty and the kids left yesterday morning. Shelly and I both feel like we have taken a long trip and are significantly jet lagged. I am very tired and dizzy and a bit down. But I know it is just a function of being so tired. It is such a revelation how we can get carried along on other people's energy—and then when it is withdrawn, we are exhausted.

In many ways, Lynn's visit was my major goal. I wanted to feel well enough to be able to participate when they came. I needed to have plans made, the house ready, etc. I do believe it was a success—we had some memorable times for everyone. I got to feel normal for a week.

So now I get back to healing and helping Shelly. This week I need to do as little as possible so I can see how tired I really am. I'd also like to resume doing some things that feed my soul, like this writing—and probably read more Vein of Gold *and follow the directions . . . I am feeling depressed and aimless. I know it is especially due to the fatigue, when I am tired I am down. And secondarily it is depressing that I have no reserves of energy. There is also a small percentage of feeling useless and aimless. That last part is worth acknowledging because I need to break the pattern of moving into action, getting busy and finding a new goal to feel worthwhile.*

It took more than a week to recover from the visit. I was surprised and disappointed to find how significantly a week of fun had depleted my bank account of energy.

July 16, 1998

Over the past few days I have been down about how poorly I am feeling. It could be just recovery from the visit or it could be complicated by the heat, or, etc. At any rate I am not feeling well at all. Very tired and dizzy. This morning . . . felt reminiscent of the really sick days—room moving, aching all over. I don't want to dwell on this, just to note it.

July and August fell into a pattern of building my reserves of energy balanced by trying new activities, experimenting. The heat was a problem because my energy evaporated when the temperature was over 90 degrees, and it was, unusually for Portland, over 90 degrees most of the time. Central air conditioning is a rarity in temperate Portland. We bought a window unit for our bedroom, so there was one room in the house where I could retreat. Command central was no longer the sun room!

My life felt busy and full even though I was home alone most of the time. To some extent I was busy because it took me longer to do things. It was increasingly clear now that I was able to work, attend an event, or tackle a project for only about an hour before I needed to rest. If I worked longer than that I felt pressure in my ears and I started to feel shaky or nauseated. Having friends over to dinner was enough focus for a week: one day to shop, two days to prepare the meal, one day to set up the house. If I wasn't careful to plan events this way, by the time the event arrived I was too sick to be part of it. It felt good to have figured out the right balance and to be able to enjoy social events and projects again, even if it took me longer.

Then I noticed something I could scarcely remember: I began to enjoy some really good days.

July 20, 1998

I felt better yesterday than I have for a long while. I am excited about continuing to rest and rebuilding my reserves. I feel full of a strong intention to get healthy. Those glimpses I have of feeling close to 100% are intoxicating. They come when I am restful and restricted in action but still they come and that's where I need to start. The cool weather yesterday and again this morning were a real lift.

Even though there were not enough good days to identify a trend they were always welcome—a vision of possibilities.

In early August I discovered something else about my new self—I could no longer deal with stress. The first sign was an event that previously I would have chalked up to "odd and unusual," but now my reaction was over the top.

One day Shelly was out of town and I was awakened by Bunkee barking at a man at the door at 6:00 a.m. I didn't answer. The same man came again at noon, and he asked for Shelly quite rudely. When I said Shelly wasn't home he left abruptly without any explanation of what he wanted. He came back again that evening. When I was able to talk to Shelly that night he figured out what was going on—he was being served as a witness in a trial, and the man was a process server. I'd spent 18 hours on high alert. I know it sounds ridiculous, but the next event confirmed the problem.

The next day I went to lunch with a very good friend who was going through truly hard times. During the conversation it was difficult for me to stay balanced in the presence of his distress—I could barely breathe. I was taking on his problems and unable to draw a line between sympathy and responsibility. After the lunch I was immobilized with fatigue and muscle aches, and I thought of his plight for days. This was taking compassion too far.

A few days later I woke up very dizzy, and my head spun when I turned to look at the clock on the bedside table. I was very tired and depressed. By now I knew what to do for these episodes: less activity, stricter adherence to the diet, more sleep. After about five days of total isolation and complete rest, I began to feel better. I was glad I knew what to do to reliably alleviate the symptoms, but I was really frustrated to find I was so fragile.

Was this fragility because I was "out of shape" when it came to stress, or did the stress simply deplete energy more rapidly than other physical activity? I filed this question away for later consideration.

After the deep release and security of the winter bed rest the slow but steady progress of the spring and early summer was encouraging. Since the middle of summer, I was not as aware of the steady forward movement. The new pattern was more like waves of good and bad cycles—a few days or a week when I felt much better or when I felt poorly again. The good days were notable.

August 8, 1998

I continue to feel I have reached a new level in my recovery. Dr. Lin agrees and she cautions me to remember that progress forward is like a sine wave and progress upward is a spiral staircase. Your body cannot adapt as a whole organism to dramatic leaps forward. She is cautioning me not to expect this level of energy—and to continue to conserve it. She got a good chuckle out of my saying I had been bored.

Daily writing helped me to get some perspective and maintain some objectivity about my progress, such as it was. During the bed rest my writing and observations were microscopically focused on hourly symptoms. As I got better, my focus broadened to include other aspects of my life, observations and emotions unrelated to illness or healing. This helped me see that life was moving forward and realize that although healing was a large part of my life it was no longer my whole life. It was possible to feel physically bad and still have a meaningful interaction with a friend, a joyous walk in the park with Bunkee, or a sense of accomplishment and satisfaction from the garden. I accepted the lack of daily or even weekly progress, but I hoped I'd be able to see progress when I looked back at the end of the year.

Speaking From Experience: Tips to Make Your Journey Easier

1. This first period of real life beyond the restrictions of bed rest was rich in new lessons. There were constant ups and downs as I cycled through periods of severe symptoms and days when I felt more energy and a new optimism. I felt better when I rested and kept activity to a minimum. I was impatient to jump into life again, but when I tried to replicate my past life I was instantly sick for weeks. Although it was hard to let go of my former life, I needed to face the fact that the past was not a part of my future. My professional life was over. I needed to find a new life that was satisfying and fulfilling and respected my limits. This is a key to getting on the path to healing—to finding balance.

2. The first step in making the shift to a new life was changing my thinking. It wasn't enough to simply change the things I was doing. If I approached new activities with the same vigor and goal orientation as I was used to, any new activity made me sick as well. It was impossible to step toward a new life without addressing my assumptions about myself—my need to be productive, successful, and busy. It took years to make the change, but my understanding of the extent of the shift emerged at this early stage.

3. My urges to retreat to my former life were signaled by periods of feeling aimless and useless. When I felt this way I was tempted to get busy, to make social commitments, to entertain the idea of working again. Every time I responded to these aimless and useless feelings by creating a blur of activity, my old response, I made myself sick again. I needed to stop my pattern of overdoing activity, and I needed to remember that periods of action called for periods of rest.

Suggested Reading

Cameron, J. (1997). *Vein of Gold: A Journey to Your Creative Heart*. New York: Jeremy P. Tarcher.

10

Vestibular Rehabilitation

AUGUST 1998–OCTOBER 1998

When I saw Dr. Black the last week of August he concluded that the hydrops, or swelling, was resolved and I was (finally!) ready to begin rehabilitation therapy. I should have been elated with this progress, but these past years had taught me that two steps forward were generally accompanied by one step back. I was pleased, but I wasn't expecting smooth sailing from here on out.

Dr. Black patiently explained the basics of balance again so I understood what the therapy was designed to do.

Proper balance requires communication and coordination among the brain, the eyes, the inner ear, and the muscles. The inner ear damage—the fistulas—distorted the communication from my ears and gave my brain incorrect information. My brain had learned to ignore information sent by my ears and instead used my eyes and muscles for all balance information.

Proper balance requires communication and coordination among the brain, the eyes, the inner ear, and the muscles. The inner ear damage—the fistulas—distorted the communication from my ears and gave my brain incorrect information. My brain had learned to ignore information sent by my ears and instead used my eyes and muscles for all balance information.

Now the fistulas were healed and the hydrops was gone, but my brain didn't know that and continued to ignore input from my ears. Rehabilitation therapy was designed to get all parts of the balance system "talking" together again—to train my brain into relying on the information from my now-reliable ears and other senses.

My immediate thought was, "Thank goodness! I knew something was still off." The fistulas and hydrops were fixed but I still wasn't right. For example, I couldn't trust myself driving on the freeway. When I needed to turn my head rapidly from side to side I got dizzy, and I wasn't confident about how far away I was from other cars when I tried to merge in front of them. Now I understood this "communication" problem and could see why I still felt unbalanced.

Starting in early September, I met with Colette Angel for rehabilitation therapy. Colette had done all my original balance testing. I liked her very much, and I respected her expertise. I now had weekly appointments with her to learn new exercises and confer with her about my progress and test aspects of my balance. At the first session, she repeated some of the earlier tests to establish a baseline before rehabilitation started so we could make comparisons to chart progress. Then she introduced the first set of exercises.

One exercise involved holding a photograph up in front of me and moving it back and forth horizontally while following it with my eyes. After fifteen to twenty repetitions I was to move it up and down vertically, again fifteen to twenty times, following it with my eyes. Other exercises involved moving my eyes from side to side between two fixed focal points, such as a photograph held in each hand. All of the early exercises were done in a seated position, and I did the exercises twice every day for fifteen to twenty minutes each time.

The exercises often made me feel clumsy and silly. There were a lot of simple things I couldn't do. I was soon fascinated by the connections (or, in my case, the lack of connections) among my brain, my eyes, and my ears and how those connections caused my body to move.

These exercises reintroduced steady progress into my healing. Each new exercise made me nauseated and dizzy for at least the first several days. For the more difficult exercises this response persisted for a few weeks. When I was able to do each exercise without symptoms, I got to do them standing up instead of seated, which was a little more challenging, but I also made a little more progress. Each week Colette introduced new exercises based on the progress I had made the previous week and the skills I had developed in the previous exercises.

One exercise was my nemesis: marching in place with my eyes closed. It was the "in place" part that was hard. When I opened my eyes I would invariably find I'd traveled several feet forward or turned almost 90 degrees to one side. This was a strong illustration that my brain was still depending on my eyes; without my eyes, I did not know where I was spatially. Another exercise showed this, too: turning my head and eyes to the side and then back to the front while continuing to walk in a straight line. At first, it was impossible to turn my head and eyes without my feet drifting to the side as well. But the early successes with the exercises showed me that it was only a matter of time before I learned or relearned this aspect of balance.

During this rehab time, I spent most of my days feeling lousy—nauseous and dizzy, not interested in eating or much of anything. Walking helped a little, but mostly I rested, read, and meditated. There wasn't much of me left for any kind of life. I never once considered stopping, though—the therapy was the key to a functioning balance system and a more normal life.

I must say a word about the nausea. By now I realized I was one of the lucky ones. When I was nauseous, although I felt like I was about to throw up I usually didn't get that far. Instead, I had the opposite problem: My intestinal tract locked up and I had severe gas pains. Dr. Black had explained that nausea responses varied by individual, and my pattern was well established by now.

When I was confident enough, I incorporated some of the vestibular rehab exercises into my daily walks, much to the amusement of my neighbors. There was a particularly flat and straight block where I could practice turning my head to either side as I walked. The telephone poles farther ahead along the street were very helpful as a focal point I could keep coming back to. At the end of the street was a private little turnaround where I closed my eyes and tried to walk in a straight line, heel to toe. I did several other standing and moving eye exercises at this same point. Thankfully, this was a place with lots of squirrels for Bunkee to chase so she didn't sit there and watch me quizzically as I did my version of vestibular rehab performance art.

One of my goals was to be able to attend weekly synagogue services again. Before I got sick, and long before the isolation of the bed rest, Shelly and I had attended synagogue services regularly. I had been unable to celebrate Passover in April with the community, so one of my rehab goals was to be healthy enough to fully take part in Rosh Hashanah and Yom Kippur in September.

In early September I experimented by attending Saturday services. All of the good things I remembered were there, but unfortunately I was nauseated within a very short time and forced to leave. Rosh Hashanah was only a few weeks away. I realized I was unlikely to make sufficient progress with the eye exercises to attend three- to four-hour services several days in a row.

I told Colette about my symptoms at the synagogue and asked for her advice. The service is held in a large room with a very high ceiling, there is an almost constant movement among the congregation members, and I needed to follow the service in a book written in Hebrew and English. Complicating matters is the fact that Hebrew is read is right to left, whereas English is read left to right. Furthermore, the Hebrew is printed on the right-hand pages, and the English translation is on the left. I have to go back and forth between the two to confirm my understanding of the words. Also, of course, there was a lot of standing up and sitting down throughout the service.

There were too many factors to isolate one cause of the nausea. Colette advised blocking out as much motion as possible and being solidly supported while sitting and standing. My brain was receiving signals, either from my eyes or my ears, that it was unable to interpret. These garbled signals were the cause of the nausea. This confirmed that my problem with crowds had a well-understood vestibular basis. The triggering environments were more than just a stadium-size crowd or a busy street with people moving in both directions. "Crowds" could be a dinner party with six or eight normally active interesting people. In fact, I found that "three's a crowd" had a vestibular, in addition to a romantic, reference. Sometimes it was certainly the case for me. The fewer the people present, the more time I could spend in a social situation before the symptoms kicked in. Armed with Colette's advice, I was ready to give the synagogue another, better attempt.

The High Holy Days begin with Rosh Hashanah (the Jewish New Year) and end with Yom Kippur (the time to ask forgiveness and make new beginnings). In the fall of 1998, the High Holy Days were particularly important because the past year had been filled with changes I was seeking to understand.

I picked up a brochure offering tips for deepening the experience of the High Holy Days. It posed four questions and suggested steps to put the responses into action. I decided to write out my answers as a part of my daily writings. The first question was focused on praise: "What wonders and miracles, both shared and private, move you to give praise this year?"

September 16, 1998

The last year has been one of the most momentous and dramatic of my life. For each of the three major events—I can say without hesitation I now see as a miracle. I left my job due to illness, my father died and I dedicated myself to healing. By far the most powerful of these was my father's death. That he was so well and lucid at Thanksgiving with everyone around was miraculous— and we appreciated it very deeply at the moment. The way his death unfolded—the love of the St. Joseph's staff, the deep respect of my sisters, . . . the blessing of being there at the end to witness the peace, no struggle, and the deep joy of Dad's passing. It was confirming of my faith and Shelly's. I felt my prayers were answered and I am humbled by the power of those wonders. I can only feel they were in honor of what my father had given in his life. The time to truly reflect, to deal with the grief and build an active relationship in spirit with my father is the blessing of coupling my healing with his death.

The illness has been a blessing in my life. On the most practical level, I needed to leave my job—I had lost balance and perspective, I had lost joy, I was taking too much responsibility. I can see now that it was the only way out for me in some ways and there is no small wonder in that. More importantly, being sick has given me back my marriage and my life. Shelly and I were both so busy we were "ships passing in the night." My slowing down drastically gives us a base and his support, patience, and caring all through the last year is wondrous. There were many options and I hope I would do the same. That so much good would come from something that is obviously negative is a miracle. I do not know that God creates what we need in the world, but I am certain that my faith opens me up to the miraculous possibilities in what I encounter.

The other miracles I have to give praise for also come from my healing. It is truly amazing how complex an organism the human body is. I am deeply appreciative of that fact and more dedicated than ever to honoring my body as the miracle it is.

This has been a year in which the miracle in the commonplace has been evident because of the pace and my ability to reflect. It has made me even more humble and in awe of the world around me. And I can also see there is far more to see, to appreciate, on the journey ahead.

These four questions invited me to go deep inside and discover the unvarnished truth about my state of mind. My overwhelming feeling was gratitude. I did not have complete understanding or perspective, but I was in the midst of an unfolding that felt like a gift. Writing the answers to the four questions provided perspective to help me see I was regaining balance in my life.

One of the other significant features of the High Holy Days is the memorial prayer on Yom Kippur for departed family members. A candle is lit the night before, and a special prayer repeated in the home as well. Even though I had performed this private ritual a few times since Dad's death, I had not been able to take part in the public prayers because of my illness. There was something about the upcoming public nature of the prayers that caused a deep reaction.

September 14, 1998

As I was drifting off to sleep I was thinking of my father—several complicated things I don't quite understand. I was remembering the yahrzeit candle we bought and had a clear sense that on one level it was an appropriate and fulfilling thing—on another level it felt like I was driving Dad away. He is so actively here with me and for me, his presence is so real, that doing a ritual act that observes his death appears to push him away into a frozen, formal realm—gone. And he does not feel gone at all in my heart and soul. But maybe that is what the candle symbolizes, the life of memory that is a light forever.

Learning to cope with my father's death was similar to learning to cope with the healing. I had never done it before; I was unsure whether my feelings and experiences were a natural part of the process or whether I was getting stuck in an emotional cul de sac. Only time would tell, and it was more valuable to keep watching than to draw conclusions now.

I was also looking forward to the social events surrounding the High Holy Days—the community side of being Jewish. It's traditional to go to a dinner after services the evening before Rosh Hashanah. We were invited to the home of one of our closest friends. The service was about an hour long. By the time I got to dinner I was dizzy and unable to figure out any way to calm the dizziness down. The dizziness was distracting enough, but soon I began to feel nauseated too and was barely able to hold on until I thought it was acceptable to leave. The measure of acceptability was a personal one; these were close friends and they were ready to understand anything I needed to do. I wanted to be normal! I wanted Shelly to be able to stay and enjoy the meal! Also, I did not want to admit defeat.

When we got home I went right to sleep. I hoped sufficient rest would allow me to attend services the next day. I woke at 1:30 a.m. and everything was moving. I was moving, the bed was moving, the room was moving. I was convinced I was going to be sick. The nausea and movement continued all night, so I never got back to sleep. I sat up in bed and watched the hours pass. There was plenty of time to accept the obvious: I could not attend services over the next few days.

The nausea and dizziness continued over the next week, this time compounded by a herpes outbreak. I had just realized that herpes outbreaks were characteristic of my worst episodes. I was forced to abandon my plans to attend the entire Yom Kippur service, although I did go to the synagogue for a few hours. There was no sense of confusion about whether I was able to attend; it was obvious beyond discussion. Neither was there a sense of frustration: I knew things like this happened.

What I did feel was disappointment and as though I had failed. I still defaulted to my "push through" approach—as if I could control the symptoms. I was slowly realizing that it didn't matter how badly I wanted something or how hard I tried. This failure wasn't about a lack of discipline or control or will. I had discipline and will to spare. What I didn't have was balance or the patience and perspective to accept my limits. I was still acting out my old patterns, trying to use my old tricks. I was not healthy yet. It was more than my brain that needed new "in balance" signals.

✳   ✳   ✳

During this downturn, I conferred with both Colette and Dr. Lin, my acupuncturist. When I described the events of the night before Rosh Hashanah to Colette she said it appeared to be a hydrops episode. We identified several possible triggering events: the eye exercises that tired me out, a movie I tried to watch at a big-screen theater, the herpes outbreak, the synagogue. She concluded that it was probably a combination of these events that created too much vestibular stress. I wanted to find the key, the one thing I could eliminate or change and thus control. Only much later did I begin to understand that I could not attend a series of events unless I had days of rest between each one.

Colette thought I was ready to drop back to once a day for the exercises but that I would need to keep doing them indefinitely. They were necessary to keep my balance system fit. She also advised me to do the exercises more frequently when I was having an episode.

Dr. Lin advised me to live a quiet and peaceful life for awhile longer. This was her calm but firm way of reminding me I was rushing things and the healing was going to take longer than I wanted. This was the same sentiment Paul expressed when I asked him if he had some thoughts on what I should expect in terms of a time frame for feeling well. He responded "It will take as long as it takes." The better I felt, the more impatient I became about achieving the next plateau. I continued to expect my version of a miracle cure.

The healing may take longer than you want it to; don't rush. "It will take as long as it takes."

I felt worse in September than I had during the summer. I was disappointed in myself and experiencing more doubts about whether I would get any better, but I was not quite ready to accept this current state of health as the end of my healing.

It was a constant challenge to find the right balance between activity and rest. On the one hand, I thought it was essential to keep increasing my activity level to improve my level of balance "fitness." On the other hand, it was equally essential to rest enough to build a savings account of energy rather than routinely depleting it. Early on in my healing, achieving this balance was like walking on a tightrope: Any slight misstep sent me plummeting. In recent months the challenge had been more comparable to a balance beam: I was able to stumble a little and catch myself before a serious fall. It was a constant vigil.

My old idea of getting well—move on and forget the illness ever happened— appeared more and more unlikely. I needed to narrow my focus to the next step, continuing to make progress, rather than focusing on the end result.

October 9, 1998

I am getting well, but I am not well. I was struck the other day by the importance of the concept of balance to me. I have a balance disorder; my life was way out of balance and now I need to assure that balance in order to get well.

Speaking From Experience: Tips to Make Your Journey Easier

1. It helped me to write about my experiences with healing—my symptoms, frustrations, insights, all of it. When I reread what I wrote, I got a better perspective about my progress or the pitfalls I kept repeating. Some vestibular patients can't write without debilitating symptoms, but perhaps recording thoughts on a tape would be useful.

2. The connection between herpes outbreaks and vestibular episodes is common for many vestibular patients. At first, I thought the vestibular episodes brought on the herpes outbreaks, but eventually I learned it was the opposite. I could have saved myself many episodes if I had consulted a physician and addressed the herpes with medication at this early stage.

3. In the months after bed rest I experimented with one activity at a time and observed my symptoms. In September I began to combine events, which caused more symptoms and made it difficult to sort out which specific event had triggered symptoms. I found that, as a rule of thumb, several isolated events separated by rest and spread out over a day are easier for me to tolerate than the same three events in a row.

4. Dr. Black assured me that finding the balance between activity and rest is a constant challenge for vestibular patients. This balance depends on the patient and their specific vestibular problems. It also can vary from day to day depending on uncontrollable factors like the weather (e.g., heat or barometric pressure) as well as the types and duration of activities. The list goes on. It takes a long time to successfully fine-tune your own personal balance. You will need to approach this as an experiment: Try different approaches, keep good notes, and see what works.

11

Life Lessons

OCTOBER 1998–DECEMBER 1998

The next step in my treatment turned out to be vision therapy.

At the end of September, thirty months after the problem started, nine months after the bed rest, and just before I was about to complete the rehabilitation program, I checked in with Dr. Black to assess my progress. I had completed the six weeks of increasingly challenging exercises and, despite my recent setbacks, current tests showed that my balance was in the normal range. However, I still had motion sickness in crowds and other real-life symptoms that indicated more therapy was necessary.

Dr. Black was upbeat about my progress. He referred me to Dr. Bradley Coffey, a professor of optometry at Pacific University, who worked closely with Dr. Black in coordinating vestibular rehabilitation with specific vision therapy.

I was relieved to have someone to consult for further assistance. I wanted as much help as I could get to meet Dr. Black's expectations for continuing improvement—not to mention my own expectations. My situation was not unlike that of Humpty Dumpty: "All the king's horses and all the king's men couldn't put Humpty together again." Like Humpty Dumpty, it took a team of experts to locate and mend all my damaged pieces.

My first appointment with Dr. Coffey was grueling because it involved another battery of tests. When he examined my vision, he found that my current contact lens prescription substantially overcorrected my left eye. Once he pointed it out I did notice that I wasn't really seeing well out of my left eye. It turns out that everybody has a dominant eye. My right eye had taken almost total control, and it wasn't until I put my hand over my right eye, like a patch, that I realized everything was blurry out of my left eye. Dr. Coffey thought this was causing motion and depth perception problems. He also found that my right eye was misaligned; it aimed lower than my left eye and was causing double vision.

After the testing, Dr. Coffey explained that the objective of visual rehabilitation was to make my vision even stronger, to create a stable foundation for balance. The brain constantly integrates information from the ears and muscles a well as the eyes. The balance signals from the ear are adaptable, and they calibrate with vision signals. If the vision-based balance signals are rock solid, true north, then the calibration is sound. If the vision signals fluctuate, however (like if I had double vision), the calibration is not effective. My vision needed to be so solid that the brain wouldn't question the information. Then, and only then, would my brain start to incorporate additional information from other sources, such as my ears.

> The brain constantly integrates information from the ears and muscles as well as the eyes. The balance signals from the ear are adaptable, and they calibrate with vision signals. If the vision-based balance signals are rock solid, true north, then the calibration is sound. If the vision signals fluctuate, however, the calibration is not effective.

Dr. Coffey was surprised when I told him I spent a lot of time reading. Many patients with vestibular disorders can no longer read. When I took a computer-based reading test for speed and comprehension, the test confirmed my abilities, so other rehab was unnecessary. However, Dr. Coffey recommended I consult with an optometrist, Dr. Bill Berman, to find the precise vision correction I needed and then come back in six weeks. This gave me four weeks to wear a new lens prescription and allow my balance system to adjust to any changes.

Dr. Berman spent a long time taking my health history because I was a referral from Dr. Coffey with a history of vestibular problems. He was sensitive about doing something to my vision that might unintentionally exacerbate my balance issues. He performed a preliminary exam, but before he made a recommendation he wanted to confer with Dr. Coffey. His main issue was the astigmatism he found in both my eyes. The astigmatism had been too minor to bother correcting previously, but he recommended correcting my right eye at this point. Dr. Coffey was concerned about treating the astigmatism because of the potential impact on my balance problems. On the basis of Dr. Coffey's concern, Dr. Berman didn't make an astigmatic correction.

After wearing the new contacts for four weeks, I didn't notice any remarkable difference. I religiously tested my vision in each eye every day, and my left eye was still pretty blurry. I went back to consult with Dr. Coffey. When he repeated a few of the earlier tests he continued to record issues with depth perception and the different alignment level of my right and left eyes. The depth perception problems were definitely related to overall vision in my left eye. I needed to return to Dr. Berman for another go at vision correction.

I took advantage of the opportunity to ask Dr. Coffey a few questions about my other symptoms particularly, the fatigue and dizziness I felt when in a crowd. He thought if these symptoms did resolve (and he was not sure they would) it would be gradual. He reinforced Dr. Black's advice to "sneak up on things" and encouraged what he called "conditioning." He advised me that, if there were specific situations I found challenging, to keep trying to find strategies to adjust to these situations. Adapting to problem situations is a fundamental tenet of vestibular rehabilitation.

> If there are specific situations you find challenging, keep trying to find strategies to adjust to these situations. Adapting to problem situations is a fundamental tenet of vestibular rehabilitation.

Dr. Berman was not surprised to see me back at his office. Over the next few months we tried a variety of corrections for my left eye. I even experimented with the lenses to correct astigmatisms, but they made me very sick immediately—adapting to them was too much like torture, so we abandoned that approach. Even with more common approaches, I often felt I was walking around with a patch on my left eye. The first few times I returned to his office I was embarrassed to show up so soon, and so often! This embarrassment soon dissipated. It would take over six months to find the right correction. I just happened to be at the stage of life when people experience a phenomenon called "spasms of focus"—my eyes were changing back and forth, so it was nigh on impossible to find the right correction. Any further progress with rehab took a back seat to this fluctuating vision.

Blocked again! Why couldn't anything be straightforward?

*   *   *

In mid-October I got a phone call from my sister Jill, who lived in North Carolina; she had found a lump in her breast and was having it removed in a week. She was understandably frightened. Seven years earlier she had found a lump in her breast and done all the recommended steps— lumpectomy, radiation, and changes in diet. She did not elect to go through chemotherapy because there was no cancer in her lymph nodes. Both of us tried hard not to walk several miles down the road of "It's cancer; how bad is it?" It seemed particularly important to stay calm and face the situation step by step—not that either one of us was very successful at this.

October 20, 1998

I have a deep love for Jill. Through the last several years in our worry, caring and vigils for Dad, I have seen her more clearly. I always loved her—but now that love is active and connected, it is vital. I admire how she works through problems—I am touched by her openness to my way—which so bemuses her. We are so alike and so different. I really want to grow old with her.

Praying brought me a great deal of comfort and insight about what I needed, which was to feel optimistic. I was certain I would not be helpful and supportive if I were afraid. I also became convinced that what Jill needed was hope, so I prayed for her to find hope.

Meanwhile, even before the surgery, Jill was moving ahead and dealing with the worst outcome: that it was a recurrence of cancer. She was preparing for next steps and struggling with her emotions about her children. Because I cared so much about her, I took on her worries. Over and over, I reminded myself to support Jill without being so empathic that I experienced the same emotions. Mostly she was her competent, pragmatic self, but she needed someone she could talk to about her worst fears. I needed to be able to listen without falling apart or sending myself into an episode.

The news about Jill's cancer got worse before it got better. The lump was cancerous; she and her husband, John, went to the first appointment with the oncologist. This doctor alarmed them by citing survival rates as low as five percent for living more than five years and recommending radical and somewhat experimental treatment approaches.

November 3, 1998

Jill called on Friday very scared and rightfully so. When we talked yesterday she was coming to terms with it—understanding that she could not let her fear defeat her, that she had to respond aggressively. She has a lot going for her—her health, early detection, the long period since recurrence, John's support, her strength, good doctors, good alternative therapists, good friends. Aah! I feel better just writing the list. I am optimistic, very optimistic. And my body is also showing me I am not at all good at empathizing without internalizing. I ache all over, principally lymph nodes and joints, and I am feeling nauseous a lot.

The doctor also advised Jill and John to seek a second opinion and set up an appointment for her with a doctor at the University of North Carolina (UNC), considered to be the best cancer doctor in the state at that time.

The approach to cancer treatment at UNC was innovative from several perspectives. As a former manager I was impressed when I heard that the entire group of physicians worked as a team. The pathologist, radiologist, and oncologist, as well as other experts, sat in the same room and discussed cases and treatment options. My experience over the past several years demonstrated that coordinating patient care by telephone among professionals in different specialties was haphazard in the best of situations. This direct communication was especially valuable to cases with some complications, like Jill's. She underwent radiation treatment in 1991 and it was not clear whether the new cancer site was too close to be radiated again. For each patient, the UNC team made a practice of ordering the pathology report on the initial cancer for all recurrences. It provided more information about the type of cancer they were treating, and it sometimes revealed mistakes. Everything I knew about management told me this team approach should yield better results for the patient.

From the beginning, Jill and John felt better about the program and the doctor at UNC. There were no frightening statistics; the doctor wanted to see more information and confer with his team. He inspired more trust and gave her the optimism and confidence she needed. He gave her hope. Before making a final decision about which doctor she was going to select, Jill waited for the final opinion from UNC. We were thankful when the team reanalyzed the original pathology report and found that the 1991 cancer was in her lymph nodes. The report she had received as a basis for her medical treatment in 1991 had been in error. Oddly enough, this was very good news: Instead of a recurrence of a cancer that had been thoroughly treated in 1991, she had an untreated cancer in her lymph system in 1991 that resulted in a tumor only after eight years. This meant it was a very slow-spreading cancer and not the virulent recurrent cancer it appeared. This gave us even greater hope.

Although there was a difficult treatment regimen ahead, and she did have cancer, this more precise diagnosis was an enormous relief. In fact, this clear diagnosis provided a green light to move into action to solve the problem. Those same feelings of helplessness and being out of control I felt during my long diagnosis period were sometimes overpowering in Jill's situation.

I spoke with Jill several times a week for the next six months. Our conversations began as heavy and serious talks about a life-threatening situation and mutated into sisterly chats about the silly challenges of her illness or mine. She started acupuncture and found it really helpful in regard to her energy level and her nausea from the chemotherapy. We also shared the *Mozart Effect* and listened to the Mozart tapes as a support to our healing. After a few months she was doing so well the illness became a smaller and smaller part of the conversation and again we were simply sisters enjoying each other's company. It was a gift to have the time to spend this way—to place each other close to the top of the list for awhile.

During October and November my primary concern was Jill. As her treatment became routine and my fears about her health diminished, the anniversary of my father's death came to the foreground.

December 28, 1998

I felt Dad very closely on a walk last week. I could feel someone there and I kept turning around—then I knew it was Dad's presence. I felt a panic—he was leaving the spiritual closeness I have known with him over the past year. It felt so much like the night he died. I saw that I needed to let him go, to move on to his next step and to trust that we will meet again there. I look forward to that. And while the grieving is not over and probably never will be—I am beginning to have some peace with Dad's death and the process of grieving. I have learned that he is not gone—he is alive in my heart, in my memories, in what he passed on. I did not know these things and they are a comfort.

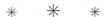

My progress in further rehabilitation was stalled, and I was upset about Jill's health. I needed to focus on something positive and constructive in my life. To do that, I started working at Shelly's office one or two hours a few days a week, setting my own schedule. He was trying to build a complicated database. Building it required someone who had a strategic overview of the business and who had good attention to detail to locate and catalog hundreds of documents. We'd always enjoyed discussing the interesting parts of our careers, so I understood the scope of his business and the overall strategy. Strategy and planning were my strengths. With my strong analytical skills I was also competent enough to focus on the technical details.

I was able to work only a couple of hours a day. I started by going through all the documents and cataloging each one. Then I listed the major categories of data. There were at least 1,000 documents to be reviewed and cataloged, so this was not a quick-turnaround project. The more documents I cataloged, the more I saw the need to make changes in the structure of the database. The project went through several iterations as I catalogued and sorted and organized. The magnitude of the effort made it easier to set a slow and steady pace.

Because I worked for Shelly, I was able to work flexibly. It was important not to feel pressured to meet deadlines. It did not matter how I was dressed or when I arrived. At this early stage I worked alone, although I always took Bunkee with me; she was always so excited to discover where Shelly hid during the day! I set my own pace, getting the project organized enough to specify the assistance I needed. Not only was I helping Shelly, I was helping myself.

The physical impact I experienced from stress on my fragile system and the continuing concern about how much better I was going to get, and how quickly, were my major emotional challenges. My only strategy was to wait and see how my health improved; perhaps the impact of stress would diminish when I was stronger. Until I knew how I was going to feel, my options for the next steps remained unclear. Responding to the feelings of impatience and frustration was not beneficial, but they were there.

January 4, 1999

Had sort of a rough week physically. Last Wednesday, December 30, I was still feeling the after effects of Saturday's party. In the evening things got worse and I was really dizzy—things moving on me. I had to sit in bed very still to stop it. It was worse bending down and still not good in the morning. I went to Dr. Lin and she put in new needles in a very long, intense treatment. After that, three hours of rest and Mozart, I was much better. Last night, Shelly and I went to the movies and I woke up at 3:15 am feeling nauseous. This morning things are still shaky . . . I admit I am a bit discouraged. I thought movies were okay but maybe I was still recovering from the party??

January 11, 1999

The episode is not over yet. We went to a medium size gathering at Rosy and Ellen's—25 people—and I had to leave. Different symptoms this time: deep throbbing headache and a sudden onset of nausea with no warning. I had dizzy symptoms all that day and the next. Yesterday was better but I was still quite tired so I called Colette and her advice was to try to acclimate to the motion. Once I feel better I am heading to Pioneer Place Food Court. I really want to feel better and I hope I was simply overdoing—that is always possible.

This episode led to an innovative new approach to therapy. Colette suggested that I find a place that gave me symptoms and go there regularly for longer and longer periods. Both Colette and Dr. Coffey, my rehab coaches, emphasized that the vision and balance exercises were designed to make me adapt. The key to the adapting was to find the motion or position that caused symptoms and repeat the exposure until the symptoms abated. I found that the most challenging place was the food court of a local shopping mall. It had a low ceiling, escalators at one end, hundreds of tables on platforms in the middle, and people milling around all the various restaurant booths on the outside. It was a hotbed of motion in all directions: Perfect! The first time I went I was hugely successful in generating symptoms. I was dizzy and nauseous within ten minutes. This is what passed as my idea of a triumph these days!

At first I tried to do some small shopping task, such as buying a card or a gift, before tackling the food court. This made me feel I was at least legitimately taking up space at the mall. It felt so ridiculous to leave the house feeling fine, walk around the food court for fifteen minutes, get sick, and come home to recover the rest of the day. I tried doing it several times a week, but it was too much of a setback, so I settled on once a week. Pretty soon the security guards at the food court began to recognize me, which I did not think was a good sign. I persevered. My tolerance rose to thirty minutes in the food court. At this point I was faced with another obstacle: Who can stand hanging out at a food court longer than thirty minutes unless one is a teenager? I'd adapted, but it was coming at a significant cost. Somewhere along the way I just stopped going to the mall. I was never able to increase my tolerance beyond thirty minutes.

Speaking From Experience: Tips to Make Your Journey Easier

1. It sounds so obvious, but clear vision is essential for a vestibular patient. I was shocked to find that my eyesight was so far off that I was barely seeing out of my left eye. I had spent so much time with doctors seeking a diagnosis of my major problem that I had let my routine medical checkups slide. I'm not sure how much worse my balance problems were as a result of poor vision, but it was clear that they weren't going to improve until I successfully corrected the problem. Be sure to have your vision checked as a part of addressing balance problems.

2. At this stage of rehabilitation, I understood that further improvement in my ability to function with vestibular problems—to resume a whole life—depended on my ability to adapt to real-life situations. Vestibular rehabilitation was based on the concept of adapting—trying, getting sick, recovering, and trying again—to more and more challenging exercises. Adapting to real life meant exposing myself to situations repeatedly and frequently until I experienced no symptoms. Sometimes I was successful, but often I wasn't. However, there was no chance of adapting if I started with symptoms or was tired. Before attempting real-life experiments, rest up and feel your best to give yourself the best chance to adapt.

Suggested Reading

Campbell, D. (1997). *The Mozart Effect: Tapping the Power of Music to Heal the Body, Strengthen the Mind, and Unlock the Creative Spirit*. New York: Avon Books.

12

A Transitional Life

In early March I saw a former colleague's name in the newspaper and decided to call him. In the rush before I retired I hadn't had time to tell him how much I had valued working with him. He misinterpreted my call as a sign I was ready to get back to work and began to talk about high-level positions I might fill in several organizations. This turned out to be an important turning point.

March 4, 1999

Quite honestly, I felt about 5 minutes of "nervous rush"—like I was trying it on. It didn't fit. I didn't even think about it for long, forgot it quickly and now see it was a big gift in my being 100% sure my future is not about that. I am serious in my goal to live a balanced life. I do want that to include some form of work: work that is a service, work that uses skills that I have to some benefit. But leading or even working in a large organization is probably out; there is nothing there for me. After my experiences, I see that the positives are heavily burdened with perils. There is no attraction, no temptation, no sense of loss as I close that door.

This conversation and my reaction confirmed the course I had been charting over the past few months based on my newfound goal to live a balanced life.

In February Shelly decided to do some strategic planning for his business. I put together an agenda with a series of questions about the growth of the business for him to ponder, complete with materials to help him think through some of the issues. It was like riding a bike! I had done this so many times in my career it came back to me readily; I had no illusions about making a big impact, but the small contributions were useful to me and to Shelly.

All during bed rest and after, I'd also been learning to draw. It started when I purchased a book about drawing, *Drawing on the Right Side of the Brain* by Betty Edwards. The book's premise is that everyone is capable of drawing but that drawing requires seeing—processing visual information—in a different way. I began doing the exercises, tricking my analytical left brain into submission and freeing my right brain to guide the drawing. It was totally absorbing; I spent hours and hours drawing, and the time evaporated. To my surprise the drawings were interesting—not Michelangelo quality, but interesting. Just when I was experiencing so much loss, and so many doors were closing, it was gratifying to open a new door just a crack. Later, when I began to read articles about the impact of creative activities on healing, I understood why drawing became an integral part of my healing regimen.

I was also writing more. During a chance phone call with an acquaintance, she told me she was excited about a book she was using to help her with creativity, *The Artist's Way* by Julia Cameron. She described it as a workbook, or self-study, and it sounded perfect as a way to explore the creative side of myself a little further—and perhaps find additional untapped energy.

One of the principal tools in the *Artist's Way* workbook is called "Morning Pages" and involves simply writing whatever comes into your head every morning, for several pages. In addition, there are weekly tasks and exercises, many of which are totally silly and all of which are fun. It reminded me of how I felt in art class in elementary school; I was learning to play again. There also are tasks for exploring past choices and future dreams. As a part of these writing tasks I slowly realized that somewhere along the way I had forgotten how to dream. Actually, I was uncomfortable even saying the word *dream*: It was so foreign and rang so false. My life was about accomplishment and production, good things. But I'd been too busy—or, lately, too sick—to dream.

My new computer skills, my drawing abilities, and my writing were products of my illness. All were things I had wanted to learn for years but never found the right moment or "enough time." I was happy to have the time and the energy to explore them. They were so satisfying in a way that much of the healing was not (impatient me, I know.) It was invaluable to have *The Artist's Way* to keep me going when I drifted or was too self-critical, questioning why I even bothered to learn. I recognized that my creative projects were the means through which I both learned new things and supported my healing. These seemingly silly amusements were a part of the balance I was searching for.

One additional thing I wanted to do was find a way to contribute to others.

February 26, 1999

We are both working quite hard on the synagogue capital campaign. Shelly is a really effective front man, the leader. He seems to deeply enjoy the connection he is able to make with folks. Similarly I enjoy the back room work: learning Excel, keeping the data base on pledges and contributions, doing status reports. It is not exactly what I envisioned as my "giving back" but it is time that I acknowledged to myself that I am doing it and it is satisfying. It needed to be done.

The capital campaign for our synagogue involved soliciting and fund raising, which are not my areas of expertise. Like any large project, there was also a need for project organization and planning, tracking, and periodic reporting. I spent five to ten hours a week preparing reports, writing articles, and making sure the records accurately reflected the pledges received. The things I knew from my former career—how to write a plan, how to run a meeting, how to effectively report on progress—proved valuable. These were necessary skills for the fund-raising effort, but I incorrectly assumed everyone knew how to do them. Even though Shelly was the one who took on the responsibility of running the campaign, I was a capable and willing partner. My work on the campaign was the piece that completed this transitional life I was quilting together.

With these three elements in place—my creative explorations, my work, and the synagogue campaign—and the rest required after doing each of them, my life was sufficiently full. I was better able to be patient and settle in for the slow path to getting better. It wasn't as if I went out in search of these elements or even that I was aware of needing these things to balance my recovery. All three of these basic building blocks just emerged; they came along at the point at which I was ready, eager to take something on. At every other major passage in my life I'd felt I needed to force things, to push myself and events in order to create opportunities. This time, with the benefit of time for reflection, I tried to watch and listen until I knew what to do rather than repeat this forcing pattern.

February 21, 1999

I have felt strong and good for the past several weeks . . . In fact I have felt so good at times that I realize I never counted on feeling this good, this strong, again. I have also seen that I did not truly feel well enough to do many of the things I had been doing—driving, socializing, etc. Now I am almost always fully there in all I am doing.

The sense of being "fully there" was a revelation. For the past several years, even when I was physically present—at work, at social functions, on vacations—I lacked the energy to join in. I couldn't engage in conversation or contribute energy to the group. Once my energy began to return, I was acutely aware of the difference in social gatherings. I noticed interesting comments, I could intuit when someone needed support to speak up, I laughed at jokes. I did not miss these responses until they came back because I was not aware they had been lost. As I built and drew from a reservoir of energy, I marveled at the richness of social interaction, something I'd taken for granted when I felt good and something I didn't consciously note was missing during my illness.

It was tempting to use up every bit of energy because I hadn't had any for so long.

March 1, 1999

I am getting much better at listening to the needs and rhythms of my body and responding. Yesterday I was quite tired and felt bad after acupuncture. I got some tea and my book and retreated to the window seat—with Bunkee of course. By the time I finished the book, an hour later, I was rested and felt fine. I cannot "push through" anymore. I don't have sufficient force to apply to make force work. And I am surprised to find how powerful just a little rest can be.

There were definitely exceptions to this impressive show of discipline, but feeling good and maintaining balance gave me visions of possibilities!

✳   ✳   ✳

Passover came in early April this year. (Like Easter, the date and month are different each year because it is based on moon phases rather than a fixed calendar date.) Before Passover, it's traditional to clean the house, especially the kitchen, thoroughly, to remove all traces of bread or leavened products. It's also traditional to have or attend a Seder, the Passover meal when the story of Exodus, of the Jews leaving Egypt and slavery, is read. Last year, I had observed the dietary restrictions (not eating leavened wheat, barley, spelt, oats, or rye grains), but Passover was only a few weeks after I completed bed rest and I was unable to clean our house or to attend a Seder. This year, I looked forward to participating more fully, to the services, the Seder, and even cleaning the house!

I began cleaning two weeks before Passover, conserving my energy and tackling only one room at a time. I started at the top of the house and worked my way slowly to the kitchen. Passover lasts for eight days, and we were going to the synagogue for the first-night Seder. We decided to host a Seder at our house the second night. Shelly's parents, Betty and Arthur, were coming, and they could help with the Seder preparations.

Once the house was clean and ready for Passover, I started in on the food. I was so pleased with myself for managing the process well, for conserving my energy for the schmoozing and the religious observance. Two days before Shelly's parents arrived, I began to notice some mild dizzy symptoms, small movements behind my eyes. I redoubled my efforts to rest and relax. I felt pretty good by the time Betty and Arthur came, and they were helpful with all of the remaining preparations.

April 2, 1999

Had the Seder here last night after going to the first night Seder at the synagogue. After all the motion at the synagogue, I didn't sleep well or much. It was the "moving pictures and flashes in my head" again. Felt real shaky also—holding my head and neck rigid. That was a 3½ hour event and was clearly too much. Yesterday I was exhausted by the time of the Seder, but it was enjoyable. It is a little frustrating (depressing) to have such a delicate system here. It is like Paul said: I have all these weak points and if I don't keep my energy level high enough then these weak points show up. Feeling a bit sorry for myself.

The rest of the Passover observance, including Shelly's parents' visit, was a downhill slide. I was not able to get the rest I needed; there always seemed to be more to do. I kept trying to do what was required, whether it was cooking, going on an outing, or simply having a conversation. I was deeply disappointed to fail so miserably again, so sad everything was such a struggle. It did not escape me there was an interesting comparison between how I felt and how the Israelite slaves must have felt after just leaving Egypt—tired and disoriented—but that was carrying the annual Passover reenactment a bit too far. It took several weeks of my healing routine to get back in balance.

These episodes were so frustrating because I tried hard to keep my activity level below my energy level. I had carefully planned the preparations. I did fairly well right up to the event and only then saw that I was using too much of my energy and there was no reserve. I was reminded of my tightrope and balance beam analogy. I had graduated from a tightrope to a balance beam last fall but now, six months later, I was unable to see further progress. My skills were not improving. Somewhere, deep inside, I continued to hope for unlimited energy overnight, instantaneously.

March 29, 1999

Have been feeling a bit down—maybe I just got too tired from all I have been doing—but I've had a few "poor me" thoughts float by about not being important. I don't really believe that and who cares? It has struck me quite a bit that 2-3 years ago when I thought, "something is next" . . . this could be it! I certainly have fine-tuning to do but this stage of having more time and space, more balance, more depth is what I want. And it does feel risky in a reverse sort of way. Risk of giving up a hard won professional reputation, giving up earnings and credibility in the business world, risk of disappearing. I need to acknowledge these risks, to feel them and proceed anyway. Not that they panic or overwhelm me, but they are risks and they sneak out and bite me every so often.

$*$ $*$ $*$

After Passover, I saw Dr. Lin. She confirmed my backslide. Even though this was not positive information, these monthly visits with Dr. Lin provided an objective observation of my progress (or lack thereof). Without this objective input I had only my subjective, often-confused, record on which to rely. Dr. Lin gave me a stern lecture about watching my energy more closely and conserving energy rather than finding ways to use energy. This was not the first time I had heard this lecture, and it would not be the last.

It was a difficult balancing act. On the one hand, I was trying to adapt to situations that made me sick. Adapting meant engaging in these very same activities, and if I pushed too hard I got too sick. On the other hand, I was trying to keep my activity level below my energy level. However, if I didn't do anything to challenge my systems I would risk de-adapting.

It was also time for my six-month checkup with Dr. Black. As I approached this appointment I remembered something he had said in the fall: that I should feel quite good, perhaps good enough to get back to some type of flexible professional work, by this April appointment. Despite my new insights about not wanting to define myself through work, the idea of feeling well enough to work was seductive. However, this was the first time since the bed rest that I felt I didn't have demonstrable progress to report. I prepared a short description of my symptoms, the situations that appeared to cause the symptoms, and the continuing difficulties with increasing my activity level. I thought I should be doing a lot better and was concerned I was doing something wrong.

As always, Dr. Black provided new information and the perspective I needed. In fact, I began to see that I was struggling with problems too long by myself. I would benefit from conferring with Dr. Black and his staff more frequently. Dr. Black indicated that the symptoms I was having—at the synagogue, in restaurants, at movies—were real and predictable from my vision tests. He was optimistic that these problems could be addressed by Dr. Coffey. I was still trying to get the right vision correction and had not been able to start the visual rehabilitation yet.

Dr. Black also suggested that the periodic herpes outbreaks I experienced were exacerbating my balance problems. This was fascinating. I thought the balance problems caused the herpes outbreaks, because they often occurred together. Dr. Black explained that the herpes raised my core body temperature, which could bring on symptoms from hydrops. He also explained that even if I were not aware of a herpes flare-up—if it were suppressed before it became a full-fledged outbreak—it could still increase my core body temperature and trigger hydrops. This explained why I continued to have frequent hydrops episodes even though I followed the diet and fluids regimen closely.

Herpes outbreaks can exacerbate balance problems. Herpes raises the core body temperature, which can bring on symptoms from hydrops.

When I expressed disappointment about not feeling well enough to meet the expectations he had set in the fall, Dr. Black stared at me in disbelief. I had interpreted a comment intended as encouragement way too seriously and created an unrealistic expectation for myself. This was a defining moment in Dr. Black's understanding of me as a patient: determined, goal oriented, and relentless. Those are not bad qualities, of course. I was doing my exercises regularly, and Dr. Black was certain the regularity was supporting my progress—such as it was. But I was taking any slight encouragement and translating it into a new goal.

I was restricted from air travel for a year after my fistulas closed, which meant I would soon be free to travel. Thus, another important topic for this visit was my highly anticipated trips to North Carolina and Los Angeles. I wanted information about any preparations or restrictions on my activity so I could plan for events ahead of time. Dr. Black suggested I speak with his nurse, Joan St. Jean, for more detail regarding precautions for flying and other restrictions. Joan once again reviewed the reasons for my symptoms: I was still visually dominant. My brain gave some credence to my ears, in terms of balance signals, but always checked with my eyes for the final determination. When I lost visual cues, I felt bad; without that final confirming information, my brain was disoriented. The brain gives priority to balance and other life critical functions over many other functions. It is normal that lower priority functions, such as memory, are often jettisoned in deference to balance. I'd heard this information earlier, but because it explained what I was experiencing I now retained it more effectively.

> The brain gives priority to balance and other life critical functions over many other functions. It is normal that lower priority functions, such as memory, are often jettisoned in deference to balance.

The precautions for flying started with taking Sudafed the night before to clear out my Eustachian tubes for the flight. Joan also suggested drinking water to clear pressure from my ears during takeoff and landing. My ear-clearing experience while walking and driving at higher altitudes would be especially important in an airplane. In addition, she cautioned me against going on a boat—one of the activities planned for the beach trip—because of the possibility of permanently retaining the rocking motion of the boat. This condition, *mal de debarquement,* sounded dreadful, and I immediately banished any thought of setting foot on a boat, even though sailing was one of my favorite activities. Her final piece of advice was to drink more as the weather got warmer, in order to stay hydrated. These tips about drinking and body temperature were related to the hydrops incidents I still experienced.

Armed with this infusion of information, I was confident I was ready for the upcoming trips. I wanted to make the most of the two months before our planned festivities began.

April 28, 1999

I was so tired yesterday I actually got depressed for the first time in months. Truthfully, I believe it is [because] I have been stuck on this "plateau" since late March—probably due to Passover preparations and family visits. This is the first month I see no improvement, perhaps some slippage. So the main decision to make is to try harder to get better—sleep more, rest more, meditate more, eat better. Trying harder means doing less. Yesterday was a good start.

＊　　＊　　＊

By mid-May, I felt better. Dr. Berman and I had found the right vision corrections, and I had been working on the prism exercises, to correct the double vision, for almost six months. I was eager to resume rehabilitation therapy. Dr. Coffey confirmed that my vision correction was good and that my depth perception was now in the normal range. He proposed that I now work on an exercise program to produce "extraordinary visual sensitivity." The goal was visual perception so solid, so consistent, that the brain's tendency to check with the eyes produced predictable results every time— visual information that was reliable and above question.

The exercises involved getting my eyes to focus at varying widths and depths using red and green cards and glasses. The glasses had one green lens and one red lens so that I could verify that both eyes were seeing at all times. I wore the glasses to look at a series of images on transparent cards. The goal was to make my eyes converge or diverge, so different images emerged on the card. Another exercise involved using a metronome to set the speed of side-to-side eye movements along an eye chart. Dr. Coffey demonstrated the first set of exercises, and I gave it a trial run. This new set of exercises was more demanding than my earlier exercises and took more time to get through.

Dr. Coffey advised me to do these new exercises for fifteen to thirty minutes in addition to the set of exercises Colette had taught me, which I now did for about twenty minutes each morning.

Dr. Coffey cautioned me not to get overly tired; it was important to progress slowly because my brain could adapt only to small, tolerable incre-ments. Another important feature of these exercises was the goals, levels of proficiency I was supposed to achieve in each time period with each exer-cise. The goals gave me measurable objectives so I could judge my progress. Until now, throughout the whole illness and my attempts at recovery there had been no measurements to tell me, the patient, how I was doing. The therapy was also progressive; as I achieved certain levels new exercises would be introduced. Given my extreme goal orientation, these measure-able results were a perfect motivation!

On the first day trying the exercises at home, I was really frustrated. I just could not figure out how to get the little pictures to converge and diverge. When I'd done them in Dr. Coffey's office I thought I understood, but whatever worked there wasn't working now. I spent forty-five minutes trying to do the exercises. Unfortunately, this wiped me out for the rest of the day, but it did teach me a lesson: I had to set a strict time limit for these exercises.

On the second day I attempted the exercises, Paul happened to come over for a visit. Paul was coming over regularly to adjust my back or neck and provide other medical insights. Mastering these new exercises was the challenge of the moment. Paul had once been a jet pilot, and he was familiar with the exercises I was attempting; they were similar to a fighter pilot's visual acuity exercises. There was a fairly simple trick of focus: You had to look through the card rather than at it. Mastering the exercises involved changing focal position. With the help of his expert tutoring I met all of my three-week goals by the end of the first week. Such rapid success encouraged my hopes that these new skills would lessen my visual dependence and unlock whatever was stuck in my brain to alleviate my balance issues.

Dr. Coffey was not overly optimistic about my prognosis. He said the exercises may not help but that, if they did, progress would be slow. I understood by now that the exercises were difficult both because they were hard to do and because they resulted in symptoms, at least at the beginning. I didn't care. It was unpleasant to get sick every day doing exercises, but it was unacceptable to live with these limits without trying to get over them.

*   *   *

Perhaps it was the new exercises, but my ups and downs in the health arena continued for most of the month of May. With the upcoming travel plans in June I realized I needed to get serious about rest and recovery.

May 13, 1999

I took a walk with Bunkee after dinner last night at about 8. It was still light and a real nice time to be circling the neighborhood. I love it here. This is really my home. . . . But more than the house it is the neighbors—who I know and love to see doing normal things in the yard, with kids, washing cars, walking dogs; the houses and gardens at all times of year; the views from the hills and the

safety I feel walking around. . . . In these past few years I have
come to feel deeply a part of it. I have noticed people and things
that I never saw before, my routines are now a part of the fabric
of the neighborhood. These are things that were beneath my radar
in my old life. And they are so much more meaningful to me than
whether I ran a meeting well or solved a problem effectively. That is
interesting because I clearly had more impact before but now I feel
more like a small part of an organic whole. This feels like a natural
system I am in.

I have been given this thing to do—this healing. I don't
understand it yet, not fully. But it gives me gifts along the way and I
know I need to keep going until I understand.

Even when I was tired or did not feel good, I continued to walk. Being
in motion grounded me and seemed to calibrate my internal gyroscope.
Being outside was both expansive and a powerful release; if I was feeling
down or negative, walking sent those feelings up and away.

I was also finding more solace in gardening, unlike three years
before, when I tried the month-long medical leave from work. I relaxed
when I realized how little I could control in the garden: It was the perfect foil for a determined, goal-oriented person. Regardless of what I
tried, there were still slugs and moles. It didn't matter that I coveted a
plant with deep purple foliage, it would never survive in my shady yard,
needing instead a sun-drenched location. There can be some comfort
in limits.

May 24, 1999

I am at a stage in gardening that is rewarding. . . . I get closer and
closer to understanding that it is never done—that it is a metaphor
for life. And like my life, it is fairly pleasing and balanced at this
point. Not perfect, not award winning—but if you look closely there
are things that speak to you.

This was due more to the magic of being outside in the fresh air than
the obvious health benefits. Over the years gardening was slowly cracking,
if not breaking, my habit of being goal oriented. It was a rare day when I
actually accomplished what I set out to do, and I found it was much more
relaxing to garden by wandering around instead of checking tasks off a
list. For the remainder of May I was really good to myself and focused on
the activities and habits that supported my healing.

Speaking From Experience: Tips to Make Your Journey Easier

1. Throughout my life, whenever I encountered an obstacle I responded by trying harder to overcome that obstacle. I devoted more time and more effort until I was able to succeed. Once I learned about the importance of adapting to vestibular healing, I tried the same approach: I did the exercises more often, or did them for a longer time. In real life, I exposed myself to more, and longer, crowd activities. It took awhile for me to understand the rest and recovery after the activity was equally important. In fact, finding the right balance between activity and rest—between trying to adapt and recovering from my efforts—was a central challenge of vestibular life. It requires constant vigilance.

2. There were so many things I could no longer do without debilitating symptoms: work, travel, attend synagogue or social events—the list goes on. In the face of these losses it was very important to me to find some new activities that were meaningful and satisfying. For me, drawing and following *The Artist's Way* provided a new symptom-free focus. When I was drawing or writing I was able to forget my limits. These were the building blocks of a new life, and these gains were deeply satisfying amidst all the losses. You will need to cultivate these new activities to fill the void of losses and keep your life from being a blur of sickness.

Suggested Readings

Edwards, B. (1989). *Drawing on the Right Side of the Brain*. New York: Tarcher.
Cameron, J. (1992). *The Artist's Way: A Spiritual Path to Higher Creativity*. New York: Tarcher.

13

Taking Flight

MAY 1999–JULY 1999

I couldn't travel for a year after my fistulas closed. June 1999 was my "release date." Jill and I were still talking on the phone regularly, and we started to focus on this June breakthrough. Jill would be five months past chemotherapy treatment and, we both hoped, feeling great again. At the very least she would have a little hair!

We started to plan a family event for the summer: a trip to the beach for our mom and all our sisters and their families. As kids we had spent many pleasant summer weeks at the Carolina coast—rafting, body surfing, playing miniature golf, playing charades, just generally hanging out. From the time we were small to the time we left for college this was the place we all wanted to go for summer vacation. This year's trip felt like a celebration of life. Both of the older sisters—Jill and I—were emerging from our sickness. Our sister Anne was coming from England with her new beau. All the youngsters, the next generation, would be there also. This was our first family reunion ever.

Shelly and I also planned to attend an important event on his side of our family: our niece's bat mitzvah. The extended family was gathering in Los Angeles (LA) in early June. Shelly and his sister, Zina, were part of a close-knit extended family of aunts, uncles, and cousins on the east coast as well as in California. This was the first large event in several years, and everyone was looking forward to it. I was unwilling to miss the gathering, but I knew it was going to be a major challenge: the crowds at the party and in the synagogue, the long freeway drives, and simply the constant interaction. Shelly and I made our plans with an eye toward creating alternatives for me—times and places to rest and be alone. This felt awkward because the bat mitzvah was not about me; it was so completely not about me that this need to plan highlighted what a major factor my sickness was in our life. When I was at home, in my normal routine, I could forget I was sick for hours at a time. These two trips, forays into the outside world, were a stark reminder I was not whole, not a full, easygoing participant.

As we got closer to the June vacations, Shelly anticipated my anxiety about getting on an airplane for the first time and suggested some training drives. We aimed for 4,200 feet—the mountain pass over Mount Hood. There was no way to simulate the rapid and extreme altitude increase during a plane's takeoff, but checking out my reaction to a substantial altitude gain in a car was as close as we could come. Armed with my bottle of water, and sipping every time I felt ear pressure, we headed off to Mount Hood. It was a long drive—about seventy miles each way—but there were no dramatic effects. I got a bad headache and felt pretty shaky, but these were familiar issues and no cause for alarm. Dr. Black reassured me several times that the fistulas were healed and as strong as they were going to be within a year after bed rest; there was no reason to fear they would reopen. The drive was a confirmation of his message: I might get symptoms, but I was not going to reinjure myself and need to start all over, which was my worst fear.

The end of May started to get warmer, sometimes reaching 90 degrees. I drank water constantly to avoid a hydrops episode. I rationed my exposure to crowds and social activity for the same reason.

The last Saturday in May there were two events I wanted to attend: another attempt at synagogue and a dance performance. The upcoming trip was going to involve attendance and participation in our niece's bat mitzvah, so attending synagogue was another experiment. Shelly and I went early, hoping to stay for an hour before the larger numbers of people arrived. I was nauseated even before our hour was over, and it took several hours in bed to recover. Although I was disappointed, there was no reason to expect any different reaction. After resting all day I recovered sufficiently to enjoy the evening event. As long as I could rest between events and recover, I thought the trip to Los Angeles was going to be fine.

Shortly before the trip, Shelly and I planned to go out to dinner and a dance performance. We chose our seats carefully to offer the least challenge and to facilitate our ability to leave at any time.

May 30, 1999

We went to dinner and a dance performance with Julie and Michael. I don't know why it got me down so much. We were in the dress circle and I felt a sudden tilt—down and to the right. The dress circle seats are located in the front row of the balcony so I would not be able to see any crowd motion. The whole room tilted down. . . . And at intermission I started to feel sick. It just seems like I have been struggling for so long to be normal, to have a social life, to be able to be in a group of people and I got upset.

Sometimes, even though I knew it was likely I was going to have symptoms, I was surprised by the dramatic nature or the intensity of the symptoms. I'd experienced the tilting sensation a few times in the past; it was generally associated with loud sounds. My natural reaction was to freeze up, stop everything I was doing, and escape whatever was causing it. After Shelly and I escaped at intermission, we came home and watched television for several hours. Watching television relaxed me when my balance system was out of whack—something about the fixed focal length or the total lack of energy expended seemed to help. When I tried to sleep that night I saw the "moving pictures" behind my eyes and could not sleep for most of the night, or for several nights after. This was not an auspicious omen.

These little warm-up exercises—Mount Hood, synagogue, and the dance event—painted a fairly graphic picture for the upcoming trip. The airplane flight was going to be only one of my challenges; the crowds were going to be the big problem.

June 1, 1999

I woke up at 3 a.m. and could not go back to sleep. In my wakeful moments I realize I am a bit apprehensive about these trips. I will just have to view them as experiments and do the best I can. I am hoping to enjoy myself and not have a setback. I feel better than ever but I am still susceptible to balance problems—nausea, semi-vertigo, dizziness, headache—if I'm in challenging situations. So I really need to ration my energy for those situations.

June 2, 1999

It is the day before our trip to LA and I'm apprehensive. Mostly about the flight and how tired I am going to get. I think I have a great deal of confidence in being able to deal with my surroundings and my life here. And I don't know how—or don't have the confidence I know how—to take care of myself away from here. The safety of home and routine are a real support to me. . . . I am not afraid of getting sick all over again. I am taking the necessary steps and the fistulas have healed. It is no big deal to be sick a few days. . . . I believe I am ready to spread my wings and take this step. And it is okay to admit that I am fearful and emotional about it.

＊　　＊　　＊

Suddenly I was into the final countdown and the preflight preparations: taking Sudafed to clear my eustachian tubes and packing my water bottle for the flight. I needed to drink to clear my ears during both takeoff and landing, and I didn't want to run out of water.

When we arrived for our flight I realized that I had completely overlooked dealing with the crowd in the airport! My anxiety had been about the airplane taking off, but I had failed to consider the challenge of the boarding area. After waiting there for less than ten minutes I felt queasy. Shelly and I located a quiet corner down the concourse where I could sit with my eyes closed. Thankfully, this first crowd challenge was as bad as it got. Except for going to the bathroom three times on a two-hour flight—I overdid the water-sipping to clear my ears—the crowds at the airports on each end of the flight were the biggest problems.

When we settled into our hotel in LA, I was tired and a bit shaky. I wasn't used to being out and about for more than a few hours at a time, not to mention dealing with a flight and the accompanying pressure changes. I was relieved to have the flight behind me with so few problems. I put in a brief appearance at the family gathering in the evening and left as soon as I started to feel sick. Our hotel was only a block away, so I could leave and walk back without interrupting Shelly's enjoyment of his family.

The next day was fairly low key: Shelly and I ran a few errands to pick up plants and dinnerware for the party after the bat mitzvah. The real event of the day was a large dinner for the whole family. I decided to stay at the hotel to rest up for the big event the next day; I knew this family, and the dinner promised to be power packed: lots of stories and laughter, which would be intense and overwhelming for me. It was hard to sit in the hotel room with everyone a few blocks away. I felt lonely and sad. This enforced isolation and my inability to cope with these normal outings was embarrassing. Several of the partygoers were in their late 80s and I was unable to keep up with them! I did what I knew I needed to do and rested alone.

The next day, I was through feeling sorry for myself and ready for the bat mitzvah. Rachel, our niece, was poised and fluent in Hebrew as she chanted the Torah portion of the week. Shelly and I were called up to the Torah to recite the traditional blessings. It is a special honor. All the physical discomfort was worth it: Shelly and I were deeply moved to see Rachel in her first adult role observing this wonderful Jewish tradition. It was doubly meaningful to be a part of it myself.

With the serious duties successfully behind us, we moved on to the celebration. It was a pool party with about 200 people—food, dancing, loud music, and lots of sunshine. Pure torture for me now. In another lifetime, it would have been fascinating to watch the kids and teens around the pool and spend time with the adults. Now I knew it would make me sick. I retreated to a room at the back of the house and read a book for the duration of the event. Except for a brief period while I ate dinner, I did not emerge from my hide-out. When we headed back to the hotel about five hours later, I was tired and a little sick but proud of the way I had restrained myself and managed my energy. I was a participant, even if only minimally.

Heady with the success of the trip so far, and frustrated by my mini-mal participation in the family interactions, I relaxed my vigilance on Sunday. An informal family gathering was planned. I decided to go to this and avoid the farewell dinner. In the middle of the afternoon I started to feel some symptoms and went to find Shelly. Everyone was just in the pro-cess of deciding to order in for dinner. He felt conflicted because we had rented a van to ferry everyone around and were the chauffeurs. If he left, the rest of the family would have difficulty getting back to the hotel—about forty-five minutes away without traffic. I was already feeling nauseated and a little pitiful, so I was not clear headed enough to insist I needed to leave.

This was one of those "executive function" times when my brain was working so hard on balance challenges it jettisoned my ability to make clear decisions. I literally could not think. I didn't even have the capability to tell Shelly how I was feeling, what was happening to me.

I retreated to the back of the house again. By the time we left, I was nauseated, emotional, and shaky. Objects moved around me; I was barely able to speak or walk.

June 8, 1999

On Sunday I got trapped in an all day outing I thought would last only 3 hours and got beyond any reasonable recovery. Into the teary stage. I am still sort of there. Very nauseous, achy, eyes jumping, jittery—but mostly very emotional. It was so hard because I am extremely uncomfortable with being out of control around others, even Shelly. I still feel weak, shaky, vulnerable. And I have not been able to eat much. That part was a nightmare. And while it was not a blast to sit in the hotel room alone, it was far better than Sunday.

We left LA early the next day, and three days later I still was feeling the effects. In retrospect, I knew I should not have agreed to attend an event I was unable to leave whenever I needed to; I needed flexibility. So much for spontaneity.

June 9, 1999

Still feeling exhausted and my stomach is a bit weird—nothing tastes good, not hungry, slightly nauseous. . . . It is a bit overwhelming how close it is to June 17 when we leave for [North Carolina]. I knew that for six months but the reality always exceeds my ability to imagine. . . . I am in one of those "down" periods when I am so sick of thinking about how I feel, of dwelling on every symptom, of spending one hour a day on exercises, of being in isolation. It is depressing. I am not ready to start thinking about "what if I never get better?" But at some point I need to evaluate what I can and can't do—or is that true? Do I just keep trying? I think I do.

I understood that my emotional reactions were a part of the balance disorder. I knew I was often depressed when I was tired and recovering from a disruptive event. Although this intellectual understanding was helpful, it didn't eliminate the emotions or the physical symptoms. The activities I now viewed as disruptive events were the basic activities of my former life.

During this time between trips I was particularly cautious about any activity. I did not feel well for most of the intervening days, so there was more than adequate time for reflection.

June 11, 1999

I feel rather suspended—between "steps" and between trips. I think I had unconsciously seen these June trips as more of a watershed than I acknowledged—as if being able to travel made me normal, made me well. In fact it only makes me able to travel—which has the blessing of being able to visit the people and places I love and the downside of more challenges and opportunities to be sick.

I scheduled an appointment with Dr. Coffey between trips; the normal check-in, assess-progress, and assign-new-exercises type of visit. Dr. Coffey was pleased with my progress on the exercises and visibly disturbed by my story about the LA trip. He reemphasized that it was unacceptable to schedule events I was unable to leave as needed. He reminded me about the concepts of experimenting and "sneaking up" on events; he also questioned whether Shelly understood this restriction. His last question—the implication Shelly bore some responsibility in the disaster of the Los Angeles event—got my attention. I strongly disagreed with his suggestion that Shelly was not doing enough to support my healing. However, it was helpful for Dr. Coffey to mention his concern; he got me to acknowledge my responsibility to do a better job planning ahead and clarifying my needs. The key was planning ahead, because by the time the symptoms were full blown my brain would have locked up.

Don't schedule events you are unable to leave as needed.

---

*   *   *

Shelly and I were both better prepared for the trip to North Carolina after the experiences in LA. We booked a hotel right at the airport and planned to stay there for two days so I had time to recover before we drove three hours to the beach.

It was another minor challenge to be ready for a three-hour car ride. We arrived a bit tired after the all-day flight across the country, and I experienced the usual symptom of motion with my eyes closed. Even after a few hours of therapeutic television, it was difficult to sleep with the flashes and movement.

The next afternoon Shelly planned one small outing. We drove the short distance to the University of North Carolina to visit the new Football Hall of Fame. My sister Lynn had visited the Hall of Fame in the fall and urged the rest of us to make it a priority.

When I first walked in the door and saw a big picture of Dad and a few of his players whom I remembered, I was not sure I was going to be able to stay. Tears welled up, and my chest tightened. The photo was of a jubilant time—a big victory—and it captured my big-hearted, joyful father so perfectly. It reminded me of the loss; I was holding him close in my heart, but the pictures recalled his physical presence. Along with that recollection of his physical presence, I was forced to acknowledge his absence.

After a few deep breaths, I went to the ladies room to collect myself. On the way I walked straight into the most wonderful photo of all—a close-up of my father and the South Carolina coach after a game. Dad was grinning his wonderful smile, ear to ear, as if to reassure me this was going to be a good experience. Those coaching years were a part of Dad—and a part of my history—I wanted to share with Shelly. We spent a long time wandering through the exhibits and studying every photograph. I was so uplifted by all the photographs, reading about Dad's teams and remembering the good times.

We headed out early the next day and drove to the beach at a leisurely pace. By the time we arrived others were already there and settling in. The cottage was definitely not luxurious, but there were bedrooms for everyone and it was right on the beach. There were the usual mini-crises about broken windows and dirty rooms, but Jill was already handling it all. I wanted to jump right into the middle of the group and hang out for hours catching up with everyone; instead I limited myself to a hug and retreated to my room to take a nap.

In a group of people—especially people I cared about—I'd get swept up by the energy of the group. At my current energy level it was too easy to lose focus on how I was feeling and get overtired. Once I was too tired I was unable to recover while I was still in the middle of all the fun. This wouldn't be a problem if I was at home and could be isolated for a few days, but this trip was to see these people I loved—not hide in my room. Shelly was good at reminding me to go rest; he could tell by looking at me when I was getting too tired. I developed big rings around my eyes he lovingly referred to as "raccoon eyes." Even though I was tempted to jump into the group and move along on the group's energy, I headed off to my room. This set the right tone for the entire trip, and perhaps it was the right signal to others as well: I was going to have to be disciplined about how much I did.

I stayed on the periphery for the whole trip. I was sorry I had to skip a boat ride on the inland waterway and a few of the other events. I was careful to stay out of the usual family squabbles that happen when three generations get together in close quarters for a week. Those were emotional energy drains as well. I did my exercises every morning and took my walks according to my usual schedule. I monitored my energy level and my symptoms closely so I was able to rest whenever I felt the need. In effect, the whole trip was an experiment, and I was watchful and careful not to add too many layers and challenges.

The day after we arrived, the sun came out and stayed out every day we were there. The beach and the ocean were magical, as always. It was very special—in fact, it felt almost timeless—to watch the new generation enjoying the sand, the waves, and the water the same way I had with my sisters when we were young. It was not long before I coaxed Shelly into the ocean to ride waves with the kids. There is literally nothing in the world like riding waves to make me feel like a kid again. I was nervous I'd feel symptoms, so I was cautious at first. After a few rides I didn't notice any bad effects. Soon I was being tossed by the waves and ground into the sand with abandon. Heaven!

By the end of the trip we were riding bikes to the end of the island, something else I'd been uncertain I could do because bikes require so much balance. Aside from the distinct pain in my derriere, there were no serious side effects. I was thrilled; I hadn't been sure I would ever have active, vigorous kinds of fun again, but this experience showed me I could.

The only new symptom I noticed was that I felt like I was rocking side to side ever so slightly throughout the beach trip. I noticed it routinely at night or any time I was resting. I kept asking everyone if they felt the house moving. It was a very subtle motion. (It would take almost a year and many more experiences for Dr. Black to confirm that I was already experiencing a mild *mal de debarquement*. My nervous system was taking on the motion of the airplane or, even at times, a car. Sleep interruption was the most severe symptom, and that occurred often enough to cause a setback.)

The week flew by, and I was very sorry when our time was over. I was a little more tired every day, and I experienced some difficulty sleeping— movements behind my eyes again—but I was satisfied with who I was able to be for the visit. It was the celebration I'd hoped for. The trip met all of my expectations: to rest, to reconnect, to celebrate health, and to enjoy my family.

On our last day in North Carolina, Shelly and I visited Dad's grave for the first time. I was emotionally unprepared. I hadn't anticipated feeling any special connection to my father there. Dad was never at Buffalo Cemetery when he was alive, so I was surprised by the impact of visiting his grave site. Both the grave and the University of North Carolina Football Hall of Fame were memorials in the sense that they evoked strong memories of my father and his life. It was a special gift to have "seen" my father in two different places at the beginning and the very end of the visit.

It took three or four days to recover from the trip; I experienced the same fatigue and low-level nausea I always did. I dragged myself into an appointment with Dr. Coffey the day after we got back and was buoyed by his reaction. He was excited by my progress both on the exercises and my activity level—the biking, riding waves, and running. He gave me a new set of exercises and a real sense that I was making rapid progress. I was nearing the end of his standard exercise program.

I spent the first week back writing, drawing, reading, and walking. Shelly was gone on a business trip all week, so I puttered around for hours and hours. By the end of the week, I started to feel better, but then I experienced another vision incident—and, a few days later, a herpes outbreak.

This was another instance when I felt I was taking two steps forward and one step back—or two or three steps back! I recognized that adapting to new activities caused symptoms, but I kept searching for that elusive magic formula that would smooth out these downturns. I ended up feeling worse a week after the trip. When I felt bad it was difficult to keep focused on the progress, because the downside, or the symptoms, commanded the spotlight.

July 9, 1999

Okay. Today is a new day. I have felt awful for the past two-three days. And I need to admit I am not completely well and ready for anything. The herpes made that abundantly clear. My eyesight fading in and out was a real disorienting thing as well. And, I admit it, I have been exhausted. If nothing else, the fact that I have been sleeping 10 hours a night tells me that. Two hours of working at Shelly's office yesterday sent me home with a blitzing headache. So I need a new prescription for patience and I need to see Dr. Lin regularly. I had thought I did not need to see her every two weeks but I am wrong, I do.

I recognize this "event" it has happened so often in the process. I reach a new plateau and I think it is the end, that I am "well." The blessing is that I keep climbing from plateau to plateau, getting slightly better all the time. I need to reflect back on a year ago. Ostensibly, I looked the same. But the things I can do now—run, drive, fly, movies, bike, swim—the list goes on. And though my impatience belies it, I am grateful for every step.

Speaking From Experience: Tips to Make Your Journey Easier

1. My transition from experimenting in small increments and then resting to experimenting with big chunks of real life was rocky. On my first attempt—the trip to LA—I let down my guard and tried to be spontaneous. In other words, I stopped experimenting. I forgot that every successful experiment involves careful planning, close monitoring of progress, recording of results, and making adjustments as necessary. I was more successful on the North Carolina trip because I was disciplined about planning the trip, monitoring my symptoms during each activity, and resting between activities whether I felt like I needed it or not.

2. Planning ahead for each real-life experiment was both necessary and emotionally challenging. I had been sick for 3½ years, and more than anything I wanted a break from being sick. I wanted to have fun, to feel normal and to forget about my struggles. Instead, I needed to focus on each activity beforehand and identify which events were likely to cause symptoms so I could plan rest breaks between events. I also had to avoid some events entirely—like large- group gatherings of long duration that I couldn't leave, or boat trips. The better job I did of planning, the more I enjoyed the trips.

3. Despite all my attempts at planning, I still had some severe symptoms. When the symptoms were especially bad I was depressed and emotional. As a part of tracking my symptoms, I observed that this emotional reaction was an integral part of the vestibular disorder, and Dr. Black confirmed my observations. I worked hard to remind myself that life was not as bleak as it appeared in these episodes, that the vestibular emotional symptoms were coloring my perspective.

4. The emotional aspect of each vestibular downturn also spurred a great deal of soul searching. For the most part, I tried to stay "in the moment" and simply follow my treatment without questioning whether or not I was getting well. I knew it was too early to reach any conclusions. But there were certainly moments of questioning: Was I making progress? Would I get better? What if I didn't? In the end, I kept returning to the treatment. I needed to keep trying to get better.

5. Through these real-life experiments and their aftermath, I saw an old pattern. I felt I was on a new plateau. I was definitely better than I had been a year earlier. The old pattern was my assumption that I was "well" and that this was the final plateau. Vestibular patients improve in stair steps, it's not linear. It is a long, slow and rewarding process. Healing moved at its own pace, not my pace. There were ups and downs but, overall, I kept improving. You will need to measure your own progress over longer periods—six months, a year—rather than days or weeks.

14

Vacation Home

JULY 1999–AUGUST 1999

The Fourth of July is always rainy and cold in Portland. Shelly had had just about enough of that and said he really wanted to make our often-discussed "house in the sun" a priority now. We had talked many times about how difficult his ongoing travel schedule was physically and emotionally; it compressed his time at home and in the office in Portland. The travel also highlighted the rainy, gray weather in Portland. Again and again, Shelly flew across the entire country through a cloudless sky and then dove into clouds as he approached home. Shelly loved to tell me that it's always sunny in Portland—it's just that the sun is above the clouds. We had talked for years about having another place—a second home, in the sun—where we could go for relief from the gloom.

This started our quest for a vacation home—on the water and in the sun. I went to the local government map store and bought all the U.S. Geological Survey maps of any quadrant with a lake within a few hours' drive from Portland. The next step was to take day trips to all the lakes in the surrounding area. Some were very obscure, hardly bigger than a rancher's irrigation pond. We felt like explorers as we located each lake and assessed the possibilities. Unfortunately, we soon eliminated all the lakes within an hour's drive; they were definitely not in the sun.

In mid-July we headed over the Cascade Mountains and into the high desert of central Oregon. We planned a drive that would take us by several lakes and reservoirs; it was a large loop—a three-day trip.

July 19, 1999

*Back from a very successful trip to Central Oregon. Successful
first because it was fun; second, because the territory we drove
through, particularly the Ochoco National Forest, was beautiful
and accessible; and third because we may have found a location
that has some potential on the Ochoco Reservoir. The trip rekindled
my desire to be outside in more of a wilderness situation. It was
delightful to be out in Oregon—and if having a place would cause
us to be out more in that sense, then I am more enthusiastic than
ever. It was a weekend of reconnection with some things I loved
and perhaps it foreshadows the future. It is so appalling how much
Shelly and I missed and lost by being so busy—and through my
being sick.*

I returned from the long weekend excited about the second-home possibilities and encouraged that the trip did not set me back significantly. I was
tired, but that wasn't unusual. I'd been unable to sleep at all because I felt
like I was still moving from the car motion. Dr. Black's nurse, Joan, had
described *mal de debarquement*, which is a vestibular disorder, but I associated that with boat rides. I had no idea that the weird rocking and whooshing I experienced after every long car and airplane trip were the symptoms
Joan described. I thought I was just not used to the lumpy mattresses in the
hotel rooms.

Shelly and I made a second trip to central Oregon. There was nothing
available on the Ochoco Reservoir, so we decided to broaden our search. We
drove around Lake Billy Chinook on our way to Bend, a central location for
exploring the high mountain lakes. The drive was long and hot—and dis-
couraging. By the time we got to Bend I was spinning, experiencing movements with my eyes closed, and unable to sleep with all the motion—not
exactly ideal conditions to search for a dream spot for a vacation home!

The next day I was still weak and dizzy, but we had made this trip to
check out the options, so we drove up to a few of the mountain lakes. They
were breathtaking, it was true, but it was obvious that the roads to these
lakes were blocked with snow and impassable for as many as seven months
a year. We also learned that these lakes were all on federal land, with almost
no private homes. We were nearing the end of the "on a lake and in the sun"
alternatives within a reasonable driving distance from Portland. It appeared
we could find a house on water in the rain, or a house in the sun but not on
water; neither of us was ready to compromise on those basic requirements.
The splitting headache and constant nausea made me start to doubt I could
sustain the explorations.

August 4, 1999

*I have felt quite poorly for two days. Of course I know why—the trip
to Bend and Prineville. So I am feeling like I have done a great deal
of work with Dr. Coffey—and it has probably helped me do some new
things—like my balance exercises with eyes closed, walking heel to
toe, and spinning around in a circle. And I am running sometimes
and active for more hours a day. It's just that I still don't seem to
be able to be in crowds, to be active for more than four hours, etc.
Perhaps I am just in one of those stages where I want to take the next
step. Of course I know I have come a long, long way and I am deeply
grateful for that. I know what it is like to feel good again. Sometimes I
can even forget I am sick. All of that is a blessing. And I want to keep
doing what I need to do to get better.*

This trip marked the beginning of a notable downturn in my health
that lasted almost two months. In the past, my symptoms usually cleared
up, or at least improved, after a week of rest—that was not the case this
time. Week after week I spent in a spiraling fog of dizziness and nausea,
waiting and waiting to turn a corner and feel better again. These persistent
symptoms drained my energy and sapped my motivation to find a solution.

This downturn ultimately precipitated a crisis that got me to focus my
energy on finding more medical options and taking aggressive action, even
though it took me awhile to figure out exactly what I needed to do.

In the heat of mid-August I met with Dr. Coffey. He repeated several of
the vision tests from previous sessions and found that the vision in my right
eye was markedly different—another "spasm of focus." But this vision
change didn't explain my current meltdown. He suggested this latest crisis
could be a recurrence of hydrops. He was working with another vestibular
patient who had just experienced a significant relapse and Dr. Black
identified hydrops as the cause.

I was so sick I was unable to conceal my frustration. I was discouraged
and disappointed to be getting worse, not better. It appeared Dr. Coffey
was equally discouraged and defeated. As I reflected on the session later in
the day I realized I was being too intense. My professional career had given
me years of practice being intense, something that wasn't as useful now as
it had been. I needed to apologize to Dr. Coffey. I was out of control
physically and emotionally.

August 17, 1999

*I need to take responsibility for being too intense. I am concluding
this is clearly another hydrops episode—probably compounded by*

vision issues. So what does that mean? I need to get very serious about drinking enough water. It is clearly a lot harder to do in the summer and I have not been compensating for that. I need to get this event settled down, get the right eye vision corrected and get back on the program. I have confidence in Dr. Black and Dr. Coffey—not just because they are knowledgeable—but because I can feel the difference . . . .

There is also a part of me that understands I need to let go of the goal—not to control or to try to control this illness or the process of recovery. To be dedicated to the process, to do all I can reasonably do, and to be grateful for each small step. As a part of my usual pattern, I got caught up in getting well, in being well. I got way down the road and forgot to keep my focus on where I am. I feel good sometimes these days (without hydrops). I am not nauseous, achy and exhausted every day, I don't have ataxia when I walk, I don't lose my balance frequently. Sometimes I even forget I am not my old self. I am grateful for all of that and I am open, willing, trying for more.

This was one of many stern conversations I carried on with myself during this period. I was having a difficult time finding something good about this particular setback.

For the last week of July and all of August I struggled to control the hydrops episode—in vain. I was floating away with all the water I was drinking. Hydrops was particularly frustrating because it cycled unpredictably. One day I thought I felt a little better and the next day I could barely get out of bed.

August 16, 1999

Words are not overflowing this morning . . . it is hard to think of anything to write at all. I have a sensation time is rushing by—of seeing it whiz past me because I can't keep up. Some of that sensation is merely wanting to hold onto summer . . . to the doors and windows wide open, the warm sun on my face, the blue-blue sky. Some of it is that it is Monday and others have whizzed off to work and I am not—and some is that these health problems do suspend time in a way. Don't get me wrong. I do not intend to be complaining. I am aware it is probably what I need.

When I was unable to keep up any consistent level of activity, my life became a series of small, time-flexible tasks: bill paying, grocery shopping, and other household chores. It was difficult for me to see these tasks as meaningful or useful, especially when they were the only things I could do. On the other hand, these chores were my principal contribution to the business of our family life. When I let them get out of balance—when they were all I was doing—they seemed onerous. If I also focused on writing, drawing, gardening, or any other activity that gave me back more energy than I invested, then the chores seemed effortless. Finding balance was an issue and a solution at all levels, not just in my life as a whole but day by day and week by week.

In the midst of these struggles with balance, I received my first official communication about my disability retirement in more than a year. Nothing about this letter was significant from a practical standpoint; from an emotional standpoint, it hit me like a torpedo. The letter forced me to realize it was almost two years since I had left work.

I hadn't retired with the expectation of being well in a few months. I hadn't really thought about a timeline; I simply wanted to make the investment in my health and feel better. But two years! Two years was a very long time, and I felt ashamed of how little I had progressed both in terms of my health and in figuring out what I was doing with this next stage of my life.

The letter also reminded me that I was on a disability retirement. On a day-to-day basis I forgot that fact and all the emotional baggage accompanying it. In the worst and lowest times of the illness, I doubted anything was really wrong with me. I doubted I actually had ever felt any better. It was difficult to maintain perspective in the middle of all the symptoms. This uncertainty and confusion arose again and contributed to my natural tendency to feel like a slacker, as though I did not deserve this disability. Finally, the disability letter was an intrusion into my life; it required a doctor's validation of my condition and other documents.

All of these emotional reactions, combined with the frustration I felt about the symptoms during August, galvanized me into medical action.

Speaking From Experience: Tips to Make Your Journey Easier

1. In the middle of a vestibular episode, time was suspended for me. I looked around and felt I was falling behind, losing ground. It is especially important not to be defeated by these episodes, not to give up. Writing usually helped me gain a new perspective and direction for the future. When I was unable to figure out a clear next step, I knew it was time to consult my doctor rather than struggle alone.

2. Hydrops episodes were all encompassing; they surrounded me physically and emotionally. There was literally no place to hide. Even worse, hydrops episodes stretched on for weeks and weeks with no relief. It was challenging to build a satisfying life in the middle of the episodes. Sometimes I forced myself to keep experimenting with restful and healing activities—such as walking, writing, drawing, and reading—to find the right match with my energy level. Meditation was my refuge, the only activity that always gave me more than it took away. Regardless of the specific activity, it is essential to have a balanced and satisfying life even in these worst of times. You will need to develop healing routines, ways to approach life when you feel your worst.

15

Managing My Recovery

SEPTEMBER 1999–OCTOBER 1999

The August crisis was a turning point in my recovery. I had been drifting along, getting slightly better very slowly. When I experienced this setback, I was upset, and then angry. Angry that I felt so bad all the time. Angry that I was drifting along so aimlessly—so passively—and not taking charge of my recovery. Angry that I did not have a clear view of whether I was going to continue to improve and what it was going to take to foster the improvement.

Out of anger, I went back to the skills I had used in my career—organization, analysis, and personal power—and applied them to find the next steps. Of course I did not find my way alone, or all at once, but over the next few months I reunited my former professional persona with my current life of healing. I reclaimed the valuable "old" skills and integrated them with the "new" skills. I emerged into a new stage of healing. I was *managing* the process rather than flexibly adapting to each new surprise.

I reviewed all my writing and symptom records. I used that information to conduct an analysis of the current state of my health—good and bad. I listed all the recent events that had caused symptoms and detailed the symptoms. I wanted to understand what my additional treatment options were and what length of time it was going to take to improve further. And then I realized I was ready to know if I was going to get any better. I was finally ready to know if I *could* get well and not just blindly assume I *would*.

I organized all of this information; wrote a document describing my findings; and took it to Dr. Lin, Dr. Coffey, and Dr. Black. After I wrote it I realized the document was too formal, too businesslike, but in this mini-crisis I had fallen back on the skills I relied on in my career—analysis and organization as preliminaries to a decision.

Here is what I wrote for my discussion with Dr. Black:

September 9, 1999

Lingering Issues

1. I am unable to tolerate crowds. A crowd can be a dinner party of 8–10 people, a restaurant, an airport, a synagogue. Any time there is substantial movement, it takes about an hour for me to feel dizzy, nauseous and perhaps get a headache. At one prolonged event this summer (5 hours) I actually experienced vertigo. After these events the symptoms frequently prevent me from sleeping due to "movements behind my eyes." It takes from one day to a week to recover.

2. I continue to have hydrops episodes. I have had at least 3 lengthy episodes this year. During these episodes, even situations with slight movement are difficult. I develop sensitivity to bright light. My ears feel full and the ringing is more acute than usual. I also get very emotional and depressed. Each of these episodes has lasted 30 days or more and substantially limits my activity and the overall quality of my life.

3. I am easily fatigued. The fatigue is generally associated with events that cause symptoms. However, even when I don't have vestibular symptoms, I become tired after 2–3 hours of any activity. As long as I am careful to rest for awhile after each 2-hour activity I can control the fatigue. This approach is a very limiting both socially and professionally. It is also a strong deterrent to travel and engagement in a "bigger life."

Recent Events Causing Symptoms

1. <u>Airplane trips to Los Angeles and North Carolina</u>: Fatigue for about a week. Dizziness and nausea from the crowds and movement in the terminals. Both trips took over a week of recovery.

2. <u>Social Gathering/20 people–5 hours</u>: Vertigo, dizziness, felt "shut down," emotional, sleepless, very fatigued.

3. <u>Drive to Bend in Heat/Glare</u>: Fatigue, movement "behind my eyes." This event linked to a hydrops episode so it is difficult to determine recovery time.

4. <u>Dinner out at a restaurant</u>: Dizziness, movement "behind my eyes" unless I can sit facing a wall. Recovery time is generally overnight.

5. <u>Dinner party/8 people-2 hours</u>: Dizzy, movement "behind my eyes."

6. <u>Movies</u>: Dizzy, fatigue. Recovery period generally overnight.

7. <u>Bright lights/Glare</u>: Nausea, dizziness. Recovered within several hours.

Improvements—Since Disability in October 1997

1. I don't feel nauseous, exhausted, out of balance <u>all the time</u>. When I keep my activity level low and stay largely at home alone, I can feel good.

2. I don't feel as dramatically bad, "as if I have had a stroke" and cannot really connect with the world around me.

3. I am not troubled by mental lapses and cognitive difficulties unless I am overly tired.

4. I sleep well on a regular basis.

5. I can do many things along the lines of balance and eye exercises that I could not do when I began the rehabilitation programs. I have also been able to do some things physically, like bike, swim in the ocean, and run a little, that I had not been doing.

As I look back on these detailed notes, I see it would not have taken a rocket scientist to figure out I was experiencing *mal de debarquement*. Here I was, an analytical person at my observational best, and I missed it. What a difficult illness this is! When you have chicken pox, you know it! Because I wasn't looking for it, I didn't see the correlation between the flights and drives and the rocking symptoms. I failed to report the symptoms in a way that made sense for diagnosis. I focused on the diet and fluids with no success.

Reporting symptoms is a critical part of making progress with vestibular disorders. What is experienced, and when, and for how long, can come only from the patient. There's no diagnostic test for "How nauseous are you?" or "How dizzy are you?", yet it took years before my observations were precise enough to be helpful. It was a tangled web—until experience and education decoded the mystery.

✳   ✳   ✳

When it came time to present this information to each doctor, I felt silly about making such a formal presentation. I wanted to take control of my own health care in the way I was used to managing and taking control of other elements of my life. I was worried, though, about overkill. On the other hand, this was a more effective action than remaining confused and relatively passive. This was a crisis. It made sense to use strong weapons.

I finally realized I needed to see myself as the team leader. The doctors were the technical specialists. They were not God-like; they were not even full time in their involvement. They were certainly committed and interested participants; they possessed the technical skills to interpret the data I provided and to suggest treatment, therapies, and courses of action. But I was the leader, the manager. My involvement was full time. I was responsible for providing complete and accurate data and for all the decisions and all the actions. When I had been sick and weak, I couldn't lead, but now, when my energy had returned sufficiently, it was the logical choice. My physical health and my life were affected by the decisions and the progress—or lack of progress.

Over the course of my diagnosis and recovery, I actively observed symptoms and pursued treatment, but I continued to feel passive in my interactions with medical professionals. I did not want to complain or to be a difficult patient. It took years to understand that those "complaints" were actually data about how I felt, important data for gauging my progress as well as new problems. Not reporting information so as not to seem like a complainer was actually counterproductive!

I began my round of medical appointments with new determination and clarity. I started with Dr. Lin. I summarized my conclusions and then asked her opinion about what was holding me back and what could come next. Dr. Lin thought I was much improved overall but possibly worried or anxious about the crowd-related events. She went on to say that although I was doing quite well, my progress was probably not as much or as proceeding as fast as I wanted. I needed more patience.

I was confused about whether Dr. Lin thought I would continue to improve slowly or whether she was saying I needed to be patient and accept where I was. After several gentle attempts to clarify I realized she wasn't sure, either. I was also troubled by her suggestion that my responses to crowds were at least partially emotional. I had considered that possibility, but I was convinced that the source was something physical. I perceived a conflict between my Western focus on the goal and her Chinese way of focusing on it. I concluded that I was asking questions that did not have answers in her frame of reference—perhaps they did not have answers at all.

My second "victim" was Dr. Coffey, my visual acuity doctor. A few days later, I tried the same observations and questions on him, with more success than my first attempt, with Dr. Lin.

September 9, 1999

Very successful medical day yesterday. Good appointment with Dr. Coffey. He had some new ideas about how to move me beyond this visual dependence. There was also some additional clarity about the possibility of getting "well." In terms of vestibular patients, he indicated that clear diagnosis and patient motivation were the key ingredients to positive outcomes—I have both. He indicated most of his patients have quit by this point in his rehabilitation program— due to lack of progress, too many symptoms, etc.—he does know of people who get well enough to resume their former life but he implied it was not many. So I am in uncharted waters, he has run out of his standard game plan but he can challenge himself to come up with additional thoughts for me.

> With vestibular conditions, clear diagnosis and patient motivation are the key ingredients to positive outcomes.

During this appointment Dr. Coffey tested me with several vision drills he used for athletes trying to improve their visual acuity. He did this to get a sense of what new exercises might be helpful for me. This was an exploratory idea, but it yielded an important insight. I performed at a very high level in all these exercises, not just compared with other vestibular patients, but compared with the athletes he was training. This explained why I was scoring in the normal range in most of the balance tests even though I continued to have strong symptoms. I had always been active and athletic. In high school I was captain of our basketball team, and the local newspaper took to calling me "Hardwood Hickey." This basic athleticism concealed my balance impairments during normal testing. For me, being in the normal range was in fact a severe decline. Dr. Coffey decided to explore this further by "prescribing" badminton and tennis.

After a few hours to absorb what Dr. Coffey said, I focused on his comments about most vestibular patients not getting well. There were many more questions I wished I had asked. (This happened frequently. In the middle of an appointment, things seemed clear and complete. It wasn't until I got home to write up the notes of the visit that additional questions surfaced.)

Were his other vestibular patients much more impaired than I was? Had it taken so long to get a diagnosis they just gave up? Were they unable to tolerate the symptoms from the exercises? What did they do on a daily basis? I knew that if I decided to live within my limits—to avoid all symptoms—that I would live like a recluse and in constant fear of being sick.

With these questions lingering in my mind, I went to see my primary vestibular physician, Dr. Black. I had saved this visit for last because I wanted to be as informed as possible and make the best use of Dr. Black's time and expertise. Over the past year and a half, through a range of frustrations and weird symptoms, he had never failed to distill the facts and recommend the right course of action. He was the benchmark, the touchstone, the "true north."

After hearing my summary of improvements and symptoms, Dr. Black jumped right on the problems and proposed three different courses of action. He reassured me that I did not have active fistulas—what could be thought of as "the hardware problem"—the tears in my ear were healed. The "hardware" was fine, but there were still a few glitches in the "software"—principally my visual dependence. All the exercises and therapy, and all the king's horses, failed to get my ears fully back in the balance equation. My brain was still primarily using my eyes for balance.

Dr. Black also observed that my symptom pattern indicated "passive dependence." I experienced symptoms when I was stationary and there was movement surrounding me, or when I was passive and not moving. This observation explained the anomaly of me being able to engage in running, walking, and biking without significant symptoms. These activities were misleading indicators of recovery in my case because my remaining problems were related to movement around me when I was still. This information was also important to future therapy. Dr. Black was just starting to work with a rotation chair as a therapeutic approach, and he thought my passive problems might respond to this new therapy.

Dr. Black also thought I was currently experiencing a hydrops episode. He stressed that controlling the hydrops was the highest priority because it caused constant symptoms and was a deterrent to other improvement. Vestibular challenges slow down the digestive system, causing nausea and constipation. Hydrops exacerbates and creates vestibular challenges. I was constantly nauseous. Most patients had hydrops resolve within a year after the fistulas healed. For some reason, my body was not handling the hydrops; Dr. Black hypothesized that the culprit was the herpes. Again, I had forgotten the potential impact of herpes.

He recommended a diagnostic test to confirm the hydrops. The test involved a low-salt diet followed by a salt-loading diet before coming in for what was called an *ECOG (electrocochleography) test*. He suggested I try a diuretic if hydrop*s* was confirmed by the test. Diuretics are often used to control hydrops when the patient is unable to do it without medication.

> One diagnostic test to confirm the hydrops is called an *ECOG (electrocochleography) test*. It involves following a low-salt diet followed by a salt-loading diet before being tested in a doctor's office. The ECOG test is performed by placing an electrode that consists of a wire, wick or spring, or sponge into the ear canal as close as possible to the cochlea. Tone bursts and clicks are used to stimulate the middle ear, where they turn into vibrations. The vibrations are turned into electrical impulses in the inner ear, which are then recorded and measured.

This visit left me speechless. I'd thought I was at the end of the line for treatment and that all that was left available to me were my eye exercises. Suddenly, here were new developments in both diagnosis and treatment.

Dr. Black was a brilliant diagnostician; all of my tests were at his disposal, and he used them, along with the information I gave him, every time I visited. It was another lapse on my part that I did not consult him earlier about my summer downturn. Although many other things supported my healing, Dr. Black was unquestionably the foundation. His expertise in my specific illness was so deep and so broad he was able to integrate conflicting information into a pattern he could interpret. I was grateful to be in his care. On an emotional level, he confirmed my instincts: I was not imagining things—there *was* something wrong! I had been impaired for so long that I had lost track of what was normal.

The new information I presented to Dr. Black was the impetus for some new ideas about my condition. This interaction was total validation of a different doctor–patient relationship model. It also reinforced my nascent attempt to manage the healing process.

Per Dr. Coffey's "prescription" Shelly and I played badminton every night for the next several weeks. I didn't get any symptoms, and we had a hilarious time. We bought a cheap badminton set just to see if I could play, and the rackets were not tightly strung. About every ten strokes, the shuttlecock got stuck in the racket head. Because Shelly and I made a habit of never competing with each other in sports, this was a perfect development. It kept us in stitches every night. We did not have any place to play other than the street in front of the house, so we amused our neighbors and sometimes literally stopped traffic.

I was not feeling any better, but I was more willing to tolerate it because I was in the hopeful stage again—hopeful for a clearer diagnosis and an effective treatment. I decided to delay the diet and ECOG test because the High Holy Days were approaching. I wanted to do as much as I could during these significant holidays, and I was concerned that the special diet would cause symptoms. Even without the special diet I was concerned about my ability to take part for yet another year. As a part of my discussion with Dr. Lin, she suggested I develop a "limited participation" plan for the High Holy Days. She urged me to outline something realistic and to stick with the plan rather than overreaching and getting frustrated.

I set a plan and followed it.

September 13, 1999

Return to writing after a three-day celebration of the Jewish New Year 5760. Went to synagogue Friday evening, Saturday morning and Sunday morning. It was wonderful to be back in synagogue; the prayers, the full sanctuary and many small moments were very meaningful and moving. I had almost forgotten the special, deep feeling I get when we are there. Even though [Shelly and I] limited ourselves to 2 hours each day, it was enough to get that feeling back. It is very special to have an oasis in this world where large groups of people are being their best—thinking their best thoughts.

I felt dizzy and weak for a few days, but I was willing to trade a few days of symptoms for the opportunity to be part of these important holidays. I also recognized the progress I had made compared with past High Holy Days.

The next week I was able to observe Yom Kippur in the same limited way—attending services for two hours each day. We also lit the traditional candle in memory of my father and made a donation to the synagogue in his memory. There was a significant resonance between my personal need to deal with my loss and the community remembrance of departed loved ones on Yom Kippur.

September 22, 1999

Once again on Yom Kippur I was reminded of how deeply I miss my father. It was like being cut with a knife to hear Shelly announce our gift in Dad's memory. At the same time, it felt like a step forward, opening the wound, sharing our pain with the world—acknowledging it is universal, not personal. I need these ceremonies and remembrances to help me heal and keep the pain in perspective. Dad would not want this—all these weeping women. I know I need to move on yet again.

I am tired and just a little dizzy. I will start the low salt diet tomorrow heading up to the ECOG test. I am still feeling a little fragile from all the crowds and the fasting on Yom Kippur as well. I am so very tired of focusing minutely on how I feel. But the alternative would appear to be less productive. It has only been by sticking with this that I have made progress. I do really hope this test shows something conclusive that is a real aid to further diagnosis and treatment.

I was learning the cost of these events. I could do almost anything, but I would pay a price in rest and inactivity for days afterward.

✳   ✳   ✳

I scheduled the ECOG test and began the prescribed diet after the High Holy Days. For a few days I ate a very low–salt diet. That was followed by a few days of a very high–salt diet. The objective was to force my inner ears to handle the varying fluid balances from the salt intake. The diet was intended to simulate a hydrops episode and remove the probability of a false negative result on the ECOG test. I experienced some falling or sinking sensations on the low-salt diet and slight symptoms associated with head and eye movements from the high-salt diet. I also felt some increased pressure in my ears, but nothing dramatic.

Because all the symptoms were so subtle I was concerned the test would be negative. If I did not have hydrops, then what was wrong with me? This type of panic was familiar from my bed rest days when I was sure the fistulas could not have closed because I did not feel any different. I'd learned not to get my hopes up, so I just couldn't put all my eggs in the basket of a clear hydrops diagnosis.

In the ECOG test electrodes are used to measure responses to different impulses to my ear and did not require my conscious participation. I sat in a comfortable chair in a darkened soundproof room while the technician administered clicks and buzzes into each ear. Immediately after the test, she indicated I did in fact have hydrops in both ears and scheduled an appointment with Dr. Black. The next day, Dr. Black confirmed the diagnosis and prescribed a diuretic to control the hydrops. The diet and fluids weren't enough. We needed to get this condition under control before proceeding to the next rehabilitation therapy in a rotation chair.

After the conversation with Dr. Black, I spoke with his chief nurse, Joan St. Jean, about the diuretic prescription and other general concerns.

Joan patiently explained that the particular diuretic Dr. Black had prescribed was the mildest possible medication with the fewest side effects. If it did not control the hydrops, then we would try a different diuretic.

I took advantage of this opportunity to ask Joan about the strong symptoms I exhibited in any situation involving a crowd. She explained that crowd intolerance was a common issue for vestibular patients and that it is difficult to overcome. She gave me some coping strategies: Wear comfortable shoes, place my feet wide apart, hold onto a seat or the wall whenever I can, close my eyes to give myself a break whenever possible, and rest before going into a challenging crowd situation. These strategies would extend the length of time I could tolerate a crowd; however, they were unlikely to provide a permanent solution.

Within a few weeks it seemed like the diuretic was working. I thought I was feeling better on a daily basis.

October 4, 1999

I feel more energy and motivation today than I have in a while. So intangible, easy to brush off as mental or emotional but I am finding it is physical. The dizziness is exhausting and literally depressing.

I was also able to get out more and for longer times before the symptoms kicked in. Shelly and I went to the opera and I was able to stay through two acts before the dizziness and movement forced us to leave. I went shopping at Powell's City of Books, a large, crowded bookstore, for an hour with no apparent symptoms. These were things I had not been able to do the previous spring. I'd hoped to progress beyond this by the fall, but it was a welcome sign I was at least capable of this level of activity again.

When I saw Dr. Coffey for my next appointment, he presented some new theories based on his discussion with Dr. Black. He explained that straight-ahead vision and peripheral vision were separate functions and were integrated by the brain. In my case, he thought the integration was not occurring correctly and that this caused my motion sickness in crowds.

Dr. Black's proposed rotation chair therapy would teach my brain to integrate incoming signals from my eyes and ears correctly. Dr. Coffey thought this was the best next step. The rotation chair therapy provided a full-field visual stimulation: It involved both straight-ahead and peripheral vision. The theory behind the rotation chair therapy was similar to the theory behind all the exercises I was doing: repeating what caused the symptoms in order to eventually desensitize my brain or vestibular system and make them adapt.

The theory behind rotation chair therapy is simple: It attempts to re-create what caused the symptoms in order to eventually desensitize the brain or vestibular system and make them adapt.

Dr. Coffey recommended that we suspend our appointments until I tried the rotation chair—although I was to continue my exercises. Dr. Coffey also asked me about the subtler aspect of how I experienced a crowded event.

October 7, 1999

He asked me about where my attention was when I entered some event like the opera. I realized that I enter the event pretty normally, feel a strong visual symptom and look down—this self-protective avoidance recurs throughout the event. He suggested a physical approach to help me ground myself—to feel strong and rooted in my legs while standing and walking. It was a powerful suggestion for me. We even talked about how to feel more powerful, less like a victim, in those crowd situations.

When I applied these new strategies there was no miraculous transformation. I was not instantly capable of tolerating crowds for hours. What I was able to do, though, was go into a place with a lot of people with my head up and feeling strong. When I sensed symptoms coming on I used strategies that included breathing techniques, stabilizing myself, and closing my eyes. These strategies helped me tolerate events only slightly more, but I also felt stronger and better while I was there. This new feeling of strength was a blessing.

I was eager to try the new rehab therapy in the rotation chair, but Dr. Black and Colette were still programming the new, more advanced rotation chair for rehabilitation. There was another rotation chair programmed for use in diagnosis only. This was the chair I had used earlier when Dr. Black made his original diagnosis.

I scheduled a test in the old rotation chair to establish an updated baseline. For this test I sat in a chair in a round dark chamber with lots of visual stimulation. The visual challenge involved various patterns of dots projected onto the walls of the chamber and moving at different speeds. (It looked like stars on the ceiling of a planetarium.) I had to force my eyes to focus on the moving dots, and my reactions were measured.

When I was tested in this same chair two years earlier I didn't have any problems or significant symptoms. That was the test for which I was asked to say a girl's name with each letter of the alphabet, or a boy's name, or a bird name. The technician urged me to let her know if I experienced severe symptoms and needed to stop the test. I hadn't needed to stop on any test during the last two years, but I did during the final phase of this rotation chair test. Although it was not positive to feel nauseated and disoriented, the reaction was a confirmation that we were on the right track. If we could create a symptom in this simulation of real-life conditions I could potentially train my brain to adapt.

Because I had such a strong reaction to the rotation chair in my baseline test, Colette and I started with an easier approach. Instead of dots moving in every direction she projected stripes onto a flat wall that moved right or left at varying speeds. In contrast, the rotation chair was in a round room with images projected on the curving walls and rotating 360 degrees, which was significantly more challenging than a flat screen! My task was to look at the stripes from various angles as they went by and let Colette know what symptoms I experienced.

Each week, we went for a longer period or raised the bar by doing things like increasing the speed at which the projected stripes moved. Dr. Coffey consulted with Colette as well, offering his insights from our sessions the previous summer. These stripe-watching sessions effectively simulated how I felt in a crowd; it took me a few hours to recover from the activity and the resultant symptoms. After four or five sessions it appeared I was adapting to the stripes.

I continued "stripe therapy" for several months until I had adapted to every challenge the flat wall with stripes was able to offer. Adapting meant I had no symptoms at any speed or from any position. I was now ready to try the rotation chair. Unfortunately, at my first visit Colette told me the programming for the new rotation chair was still unfinished and that it might be several weeks or even several months before it was ready to be used in the therapy. I was not disappointed about the delay because I was not feeling very well and my vision was fluctuating again.

As it turned out, there were some other challenges ahead that had nothing to do with stripes on the wall or rotating chairs.

Speaking From Experience: Tips to Make Your Journey Easier

1. Taking control of my vestibular healing was a huge positive step, and I'm not sure why it took me so long. For three and a half years I had been too passive and expected my doctors to solve every problem. All of a sudden I saw that I lived with the symptoms every minute. I was intimately familiar with the consequences of all my activities every hour of every day, whereas my doctors saw me, at most, an hour a

month. This time exposure alone dictated that I act more as a leader, take charge. Being in charge meant I was more organized: I planned for doctor's appointments by analyzing the symptom tracking I did daily, noting areas of progress and areas of concern. I also became more of an active problem solver. I kept notes of every doctor's visit and reread the notes as a basis for informal experiments I could report on at each visit: Which strategy lessened symptoms? Which approach increased length of time I could tolerate events? I also kept a running list of questions and developed a list of key questions for each appointment.

2. I'm not sure why I felt so silly in my first attempts to manage my healing. I think it's because I had a set of preconceived notions about what you do when you're a medical patient, and most of those notions involved being submissive, following direction, and being respectful of the delivered wisdom of doctors. This was my error. Each of my doctors encouraged greater participation and leadership. In fact, they were energized by my focus and aided by my insights. This is a key insight for all patients: We need to become our own advocates and actively engage in our treatment. Taking charge is essential for vestibular patients, given the complications of sorting out the various disorders and the deeply individual nature of the symptoms.

3. As I stepped up to take a lead role in my treatment, I took my symptom tracking to a new level as well. I developed computer forms that listed all my common symptoms, and I tracked the severity daily. I tried, wherever possible, to associate the symptoms with an activity, or heat or rain, or a herpes outbreak. I wrote down my daily activities in a separate calendar. I also periodically summarized the symptom information to assess my progress. I still wasn't confident that my tracking was precise or accurate, but the only way to get batter at it was to keep doing it. Without it I had no data, no contribution.

4. I must say a word about getting better, getting well. My vestibular problems were complicated: I had multiple problems in both ears. These complications created greater challenges for diagnosis and treatment. It was this subset of "complicated" patients who were referred to Dr. Coffey. When Dr. Coffey told me he didn't see many vestibular patients who got well, in the traditional sense, he was talking about complicated cases such as mine. Many vestibular patients do get well.

16

Life's Ups and Downs

NOVEMBER 1999–DECEMBER 1999

Between going to stripe therapy and recovering from the aftereffects, I was working on a new project for Shelly, who was in a bind about a project to refine and improve performance standards for an airport client. He had developed several previous versions and had hired consultants to provide additional technical information on specific areas such as standards for food service in airport restaurants (a field that obviously was wide open!). Putting all the information together was a time-consuming task, and he had no time. I had spent the last three years of my career doing pretty much exactly what needed to be done here, that is, creating measurable performance standards. This performance standard project was appealing; it allowed me to make use of my electric utility experience in a new arena: airport shopping and dining.

Week after week, I worked no more than two hours a day on my own schedule, for as many as three days a week. I organized and compiled a mountain of information. I needed to make informed recommendations about what to include and what to omit, how to make the standards measurable, and where new standards were needed. I enjoyed figuring out how to break the project into manageable pieces. I was grateful that I was able to work at my own pace. In fact, Shelly was so busy he was unable to review any interim work. I took on the project thinking I was simply doing the preparations and he was going to take the raw materials and put together the final report. As I became immersed in the project, I realized how busy Shelly was and knew I needed to finish the project, to make it into a document ready to be handed to the client.

I began to write. As I began, I discovered a significant number of missing pieces. When I came to one of the missing pieces I sat back and imagined what the right approach should be and wrote it in as much detail as possible. To my great surprise I began to have fun writing the workbook. Filling in the gaps required creative leaps like those I experienced when I was drawing.

I'd stopped drawing much over the summer. When I felt better and the weather forced me inside, I picked up my pencil and started again. I was impatient (when was I not?) with my progress and had a difficult time figuring out what to draw. I decided to try a few longer studies, drawings that involved several stages and perspectives on one subject. I bought a book of photographs of dancers because I was interested in drawing figures in motion. The photographs captured dancers when they were airborne and portrayed them as gymnastic angels. This was the nudge I needed to get interested again.

Meanwhile, in early October a new development arose in our search for a vacation house on a lake in the sun. Shelly and I had abandoned our attempt to find a lake and decided to check out property along the Deschutes River, just south of Bend. We had visited Bend in the summer but had focused on the high mountain lakes, so we were unfamiliar with this property on the river.

Shelly was traveling extensively again, so we were not able to get over to Bend and check out the new alternatives until late October. When we were finally able to make the trip, it was on a short turnaround because of Shelly's flight schedule, and we shopped until we dropped; we looked at seventeen houses in one day! One house in particular, right on the river, was very near to what we wanted. It was on a big lazy bend in the river with a large marsh filled with flocks of ducks and geese. There were even photos of a winter elk herd feeding along the frozen marsh. The water was visible from every room in the house. It was bright and sunny, right next to the river. As we drove the three-plus hours home, we discussed the house and decided to make an offer.

I knew taking the round trip in one day was way too much of a stimulus, but sometimes there is no alternative. When Shelly flew out the next day I got into bed. The dizziness and nausea had almost stopped by the time he got home five days later.

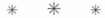

My mother had not been feeling well. For almost six months, ever since her Oregon visit last spring, she'd had a string of annoying flu bouts and infections. It was nothing serious, but it took her doctors a long time to figure out what was going on. As a result, she felt poorly for a long time.

Mom had been such a great companion when I was unable to travel; I wanted to return the favor and visit her when she did not feel like flying across the country. Shelly and I scheduled a trip for early November.

The night before we left, we went to a small event in the neighborhood. As we walked back in the door, my sister Lynn called. The first words out of her mouth were "Mom is OK." I was confused rather than reassured because we had missed an earlier message telling us Mom had fallen and broken her hip and wrist. Lynn was calling now to let me know Mom was through surgery to put a pin in her hip and that she was doing well.

My mother was 78—a very young 78. I thought of her as more of a sister than my mother; she was active, an intrepid traveler and always learning new things. Her most recent focus was the computer and the Internet. She was the one who had taught me how to manage and track our investments on the computer years earlier. Even though she had not been feeling well for six months, she was usually strong and healthy. I remembered when Dad started to fail, and I was reassured when I saw none of those same signs from my mother. A broken hip and wrist sounded very serious; I'd heard many stories about broken hips being the "beginning of the end" for elderly people. None of those images fit with what I knew of my mother. I was relieved we were getting on the plane in less than twelve hours.

I was into emotional overreaction before I even got off the phone with Lynn, and it didn't stop the whole week we were in North Carolina. It was as if I thought the intensity of my emotions would somehow weight the balance in favor of my mother's healing. I was totally out of control. It took all day to fly to North Carolina, but after our flight landed we drove straight to the hospital and were able to see Mom at about 8:00 p.m. She looked very weak and tired, which is not surprising given that she'd emerged from surgery less than twenty-four hours before. However, even weak and tired she was a sight for sore eyes. All the horrible deterioration I'd imagined was put to rest. This was still my mother: smart, alert, and strong.

Once we were reassured, Shelly and I went back to Mom's house to spend the night. This was the first time I'd been in my mother's house without her. It was unbelievably lonely. Her absence was too suggestive of a time when she would no longer be alive, and I fought that image fiercely. The moment we walked in, the phone rang and, oddly, it was Shelly's sister calling from Los Angeles. His Uncle Julie, his favorite uncle, had died unexpectedly the night before. Shelly booked a flight to New York to attend the funeral the next day. As a last action of the day Shelly checked our messages on the home phone and found out our offer on the vacation house had fallen through because the sellers could not meet the contingency. At this point that didn't matter at all.

I was unable to sleep that night—partly from the flight and mostly from the emotion. After getting up at 5:00 a.m. to say goodbye to Shelly, I was not in great physical shape. Already I was watching myself do the very things that undermined my balance and health. All of my calm resolve not to get swept up in the energy but to stay aware of how I was feeling—to protect my balance—was nowhere to be found. I tried my usual techniques, but nothing helped, so I gave up and went to visit Mom.

Mom bounced back almost miraculously. She was apologetic about ruining our visit and laughed at her stupidity in falling. It turned out she called Lynn after she fell because she thought she had broken her wrist. Lynn's husband, Russ, responded to her call, and she insisted on walking to the car and into the hospital—with what turned out to be a broken hip! She'd waited about eight hours for surgery because her condition was too unstable earlier in the day. By the time I arrived that second morning she was learning how to transfer in and out of bed with a walker; this was no small feat given the broken wrist. Within a day she was strolling up and down the hall with the walker. It was quickly obvious she was going to be fine.

No matter how fabulous Mom was doing she could not go home alone in a week. We needed to find a place for her to stay, perhaps for as long as three months. The next few days were a blur of errands and chores to get Mom set up for a month in a nearby nursing facility. (She did great. She came home a week early!) During the entire visit Shelly kept reminding me that I was running on adrenaline, and every time he reminded me I agreed with him. But I couldn't stop.

November 29, 1999

It was not good that I could not stop the adrenaline "push through," I went several steps ahead and let it upset me; I did not protect myself at all. So when I got home I felt awful. Turns out I had herpes and the flu. It is almost two weeks later and the flu is subsiding but I am having a second herpes episode.

I want to learn from this. It is very parallel to worrying about things you can't affect—this overly emotional, adrenaline-fueled reaction to events that have not occurred. It is pretty clear that my health is improving. But I feel I am simply decked by emotion. It totally wipes me out to go through an experience like the last [North Carolina] trip. And I am so readily completely fatigued, not entirely dead and flat but real tired, unmotivated. I don't know that the chronic fatigue is not still with me. Perhaps, I need to address that a bit more actively. Meanwhile, I am getting better and determined not to abandon balance at the first whistle of crisis.

When Shelly and I returned from North Carolina we formally withdrew our offer on the house in Bend. It was well into winter, and it was going to be difficult to find a vacation home in December. Just out of curiosity, I went to the Web site where I'd found the initial properties to see if there were any new offerings. There was one new listing that looked perfect: right on the river, just the right size, and in our price range. Shelly called the Realtor and set up an appointment to visit the next weekend.

We both knew immediately this was the right house for us. Because of our previous experience we knew all the questions to ask and had even prearranged an appointment with the local planning department. This house, like the previous house, was right on a wild and scenic river, so there were restrictions on new construction as well as remodeling existing homes. The planner's answers confirmed that we would be able to make the changes we wanted, and on our long drive home we discussed the offer we would make.

Our offer was accepted immediately, and we began the blizzard of paperwork to get a mortgage and close on the purchase before the end of the year. We also faced the task of furnishing a totally empty house from two hundred miles away. We started to spend weekends in mattress and furniture stores figuring out what we needed and who was able to make deliveries to Bend from Portland. These were not the most beneficial places for me to spend time; I got dizzy and tired frequently on these trips. I knew both the shopping and the dizziness were only temporary.

Between the paperwork and the endless shopping I was still able to get in some relaxing and fun activities. Shelly was traveling for business during the week, so I was alone a great deal. His birthday was coming up, and I decided to draw something for him with colored pencils. I found a photo of an old truck—the same model he had owned years ago—and started slowly working in secret. It was always helpful to have a purpose and a deadline; I was having a hard time motivating myself to keep drawing with no real purpose.

December 13, 1999

I am also drawing—or trying to—it is a gift for Shelly that I want to be a surprise. It's my first color pencil attempt and I can see that I have learned some things. I am able to just use the drawing book and follow directions—directions that were unintelligible several years ago. And soon I will crack open the painting book.

> *We are also buying a cabin in Bend. It is a much nicer place than the first one—sunnier, closer to the river. All of these things feel like new beginnings. Not, "down the road," still unclear about direction—but starting out.*

It was the end of the calendar year—my second year of recovery—and I reflected on my experience. My problems were becoming manageable; I understood them because they were familiar. I was developing strategies to cope with them. The downside of this new stage was slower progress. The main advantage was the predictability in my daily life: I could feel good alone, or I could try something that challenged me and made me feel bad for a period of time. These were choices I made every day with at least some sense of the likely outcome. The other advantage was long term: I was managing the direction and course of my recovery. I was responsible for the medical choices and the life choices. I recognized my physical limits, but I was not at the mercy of them.

January 1, 2000

> *As we begin this New Year I am confident I am on my path. I am excited about the painting and writing. I am pleased with how far I have come in healing and looking forward to more progress. I see that I need to keep doing the exercises diligently and I believe I need to start doing the same for strength and flexibility. It is satisfying to have hopes and dreams, to believe in possibilities. I'm so deeply grateful for this life, this world, for Shelly, our family, our friends, . . . the park, the neighborhood. A transition is maturing and gathering speed for me. I need to let the transition happen and not accelerate the pace of my life. I don't know if I will ever have the ability to move as quickly, to take the stress, to keep up the pace. And I am not even sure I would place any priority on having the ability.*

There was still the promise of additional therapy, the hope of further progress, and the desire to push against my limits. I felt I was on a journey.

Speaking From Experience: Tips to Make Your Journey Easier

1. Recovery from a vestibular disorder involves adapting through therapy. It also involves adapting to life. Because the vestibular system adapts through repetition and desensitization, the activities I repeated most

often caused fewer and fewer symptoms as time went on. On the flip side, activities I only repeated on a monthly or even weekly basis were much more difficult to adapt to. This becomes the challenge of the healing process, to widen the circle of activities and carve out a more expansive life.

2. Another part of the closely monitored life I was building involved dealing effectively with stress. I had noticed the immediate negative impacts of stress on my balance almost a year earlier. When my mother broke her hip I fell victim to stress again; however, this time I was able to see at least a part of what I was doing to make the situation worse. Under stress, I abandoned my control. I stopped making choices about what activities I could do and for how long. My mother seemed more important, a higher priority. As I looked back on the events, I saw that this only made things more difficult for me and didn't help my mother. Avoid stressful situations whenever you can, and when you need to involve yourself don't forget to watch your balance of activity and rest. Keep planning.

17

Rotation Therapy

JANUARY 2000–OCTOBER 2000

It was the start of the third year of my healing. My list of health issues dwindled to three basic problems: fluctuating vision, periodic hydrops episodes, and motion sickness in crowds. Early in the year, this list went down to two items, because my optometrist found the right correction, and the fluctuations in my vision ended. Resolving my vision problem opened the way to further improvement from the rotation chair advanced therapy, which technically is called *visual suppression therapy*. The rotation chair was my now my last, best hope to resolve the motion sickness and crowd-related symptoms.

I experienced motion sickness in crowds as small as those in waiting rooms or at dinners with another couple at home. Once I understood that this was related to peripheral vision, I developed and tested various strategies. In waiting rooms I experimented with reading, pulling the magazine up to my nose to block out peripheral motion. I wore sunglasses. I sat in corners, staring at the wall. I tried any and every approach to block out movement in my peripheral vision. If I were able to sit closely facing a wall, or if I simply closed my eyes, I could tolerate a crowd. If I couldn't, after thirty to forty-five minutes I was well down the road of increasing symptoms: dizziness, headache, nausea, and muscle aches. The longer I remained in the situation that was causing symptoms, the more significant the symptoms became. I was living a life of relative isolation and often able to forget I was not totally well. Every time I was reminded of my limits, it made me sad and determined to keep trying to solve the problem.

I noticed consistent symptoms from each trip Shelly and I were making to Bend to our new vacation home every few weeks. For the past year, I'd referred to these symptoms as "movements behind my eyes." One trip was especially difficult because we traveled through a snowstorm for four hours. When the movements started that night it was obvious they were not behind my eyes; *I* was the one moving. I felt like I was moving through the snowstorm just as we had been on the drive. Shelly and I started to experiment with different cars, driving at different times (morning, afternoon, evening), driving into the sun, driving away from the sun, and stopping more frequently. It appeared easiest for me in the biggest cars, the ones with the softest suspension, and the ones highest off the road. These efforts helped somewhat, but even with all that there was a strong correlation between how much movement I felt after the trip and how tired I was when I began the trip. Rest and maintaining balance continued to be important, but these episodes were evidence of remaining problems.

During my next appointment with Dr. Black I reported these developments. When I told him about feeling movement after car or plane trips, he suspected I was experiencing *mal de debarquement*. My nervous system was adapting to the motion of the car or the plane. It's like the swaying, unbalanced sensation you have when you step off a boat after a few hours, but in my case the movement didn't stop for several hours.

The diagnosis of *mal de debarquement* explained the symptoms I experienced as long ago as the beach trip in 1998 when the house felt like it was rocking. It also explained the "movement behind my eyes" I felt after most of the drives to central Oregon. These drives were fundamental to diagnosing the condition because there were no other contributing factors present (e.g., the crowd motion when I flew on an airplane.) The snowstorm clinched the diagnosis because I actually saw the movement long after the drive was over rather than just feeling some vague movement I was unable to describe. One very confusing element of *mal de debarquement* is that symptoms don't develop until at least an hour after the drive or flight.

My list of problems had increased to three again: motion sickness in crowds, hydrops, and now *mal de debarquement*. This was a new concern, and it did not sink in immediately—or, more accurately, it did not rise to the top of my list. I was still most concerned about the motion sickness in crowds because this had the most limiting effect on my daily life. The rotation chair therapy remained the next logical step, but the program was not yet functioning properly so there was no choice but to wait.

During this appointment I also asked Dr. Black if there was any medication I could take to make the drives and crowd events easier. I wanted something I could take before an event I knew was going to cause symptoms. I'd survived my last year of work with periodic low doses of diazepam and wondered if that was a possibility. Dr. Black did not approve of this medication for my condition. Although it did block the effects that resulted in motion sickness, it caused a decrease in vestibular function by disrupting my brain's ability to adapt, and it was addictive.

Dr. Black described a range of different medications, none of which had been consistently successful for other patients. He prescribed a medication that addressed the motion sickness and still allowed my brain to adapt. Although the medication was unlikely to remove the symptoms entirely, it might increase my tolerance for the challenging crowd situations (although we eventually concluded it did not have that affect for me). I was thinking ahead to the next semiannual family trips to North Carolina and Los Angeles and hoped medication would make the aftereffects of the flights more tolerable.

> Medication is unlikely to remove the symptoms entirely, but it can be helpful for some people.

Before there was further progress there was a minor setback.

After the North Carolina trip in November, a double herpes outbreak convinced me I needed to take a daily medication to prevent the outbreaks; they were occurring too frequently. I also remembered that Dr. Black thought the herpes outbreaks were one of the things causing the hydrops episodes. I began to take daily medication for herpes, in addition to the diuretic I was already taking for hydrops. But nothing was ever straightforward. In January, I began to have what felt like heart palpitations. When I called Joan, in Dr. Black's office, she scheduled a blood test and advised me to schedule a physical.

The results of a routine blood test showed elevated potassium levels, which likely were causing the palpitations, so I stopped the diuretic immediately. Summer was the most difficult time with hydrops; it was harder to drink enough water in the heat. Because it was now only early spring, I had a few months to see if I would have problems with hydrops in more easily controlled situations. I decided to try medicating only the herpes for a while.

This was a pragmatic, not an emotionally loaded, appointment with Dr. Black. I didn't have any hopes that could be crushed. I brought in data. He analyzed them. We devised a next step. We were simply managing the process of searching for a solution. This was my new job. This was my new business.

* * *

My first session with the long-awaited rotation chair came in May. I looked forward to starting, but I was determined not to hope for a miracle, a breakthrough, only to be disappointed yet again.

Dr. Black had been awarded a grant to study the use of the rotation chair for rehabilitation—an extension of its current use for diagnosis. I was the first patient to participate in this research project. Dr. Black and his chief rehabilitation staff member, Colette, had weekly consultations on the correct protocol for treatment. Despite my new pragmatism, I was aware that this was the last stop. There were no promising approaches on the horizon if this one failed.

Rotation chair therapy involved sitting in a special chair inside a round chamber in complete darkness. The chair did not move during the therapy. Stars or dots were projected onto the walls and moved around in different directions—one minute to the right and then one minute to the left. Movement of the dots around the circular room provided the full-field visual stimulation I needed to integrate my peripheral vision with my straight-ahead vision. One set lasted four minutes. The goal was to adapt to the motion and increase the number of sets. Adapting meant being able to do a set with no symptoms—nausea, dizziness, headache, other body aches—either during or after the session. First prize for adapting was adding another set and starting the adaptation again!

We started with one session a week. My first anxiety was whether I could adapt at all—a familiar fear of failure I experienced consistently.

May 8, 2000

I did my third rotation therapy with Colette today. I am now able to tolerate it for 20 minutes. It made me quite sick and I have felt achy and emotional ever since . . . plus slightly nauseous now six hours later. So I am steadily able to tolerate more. I hope this works and I hope whatever emerges as the next problem will be less limiting or take a shorter time to address. I'm not sure I'd choose radically different activities but I'd like to have the choice.

After trying one session a week for a month, my progress was extremely slow. Colette decreased the duration to twelve minutes, three sets of four minutes apiece rather than five sets, and increased my therapy from one session a week to three.

June 3, 2000

This week was three rotation chair sessions: Tuesday, Wednesday, and Friday. I was dizzy 4 to 6 hours after the Tuesday sessions. I felt immediate ear pressure and a slight headache after Wednesday

*but perhaps I was less dizzy for less long. After Friday I was not
immediately dizzy but I had a slight headache. I woke up with
lots of movement at 4:30 a.m. with my eyes closed. Feel fine today.
As opposed to hoping this therapy works, I feel more like I will be
amazed if it works. The dizziness in crowds seems like a fact of life.*

Because this was a research project as well as rehabilitation, we tried
many different approaches. We experimented with frequency—one, two,
or three times a week. We picked different starting points—three sets, two
sets, one set. Later in the summer, we increased the speed of the rotating
dots. All of these variations were designed to facilitate adaptation in the
therapy and, we hoped, more broadly in my life.

I kept notes of my progress and my symptoms after every session.
Within a short while therapy was the central feature of my life. I was either
about to go to therapy, just back from therapy, recovering from therapy, wak-
ing up in the middle of the night "moving" and remembering therapy, or
writing down my symptoms. My life was consumed by therapy, but the good
news appeared to be that I was better able to adapt with frequent sessions,
and I was steadily adapting to more and more time. Dr. Black set a goal of
eight sets, or thirty-two minutes. When I achieved this goal we were going to
reassess my program.

In the edges around my therapy and recovery, I tried to enjoy the summer, go to synagogue, and explore the pleasures of our new vacation home.

June 11, 2000

*We went to synagogue for two hours. It was our friend's son's Bar
Mitzvah. I had taken my medication so I could make it for longer—
and 2 hours is a record of sorts. It was a pleasure to see so many
folks we had not seen in awhile. I look back with a real sense of loss
at those weeks when we went to synagogue regularly. Anyway, we
left after two hours and I soon saw it was too much. Came home and
rested, actually took a nap.*

*The next day we went to a dance event with Ellen and Rosy—
dinner first. I took the medication for that also. Dinner was fine but
we had to leave at intermission of the dance. It was a local company—
really fun, humorous, great music. I was really enjoying it and it made
me feel like crying to leave. Poor Shelly! I am really quite limited.
Who in the hell do I think I am writing about it being over? There are
still times it feels like a nightmare or some sort of punishment. It is
depressing to be so limited. I guess I had thought the medication would
work better—or I at least thought I could sleep it off and feel fine today.*

There were dramatic disappointments, but there were also small cele-brations—visits with family when I sometimes felt good enough to forget for awhile that I was sick, strenuous hikes in the mountains, a few movies with no symptoms. When you lower the bar, a "normal" day is easier to achieve. I was generally able to manage my life and my activities to avoid serious episodes. What I didn't see was a significant improvement in my ability to tolerate crowds as I adapted to greater time exposure in the rota-tion therapy, but the therapy was not finished.

The therapy made me contort in surprising ways. Colette explained that exposure to vestibular challenges caused co-contractions: The brain involuntarily contracts the muscles around joints to keep the body more stable. To keep myself from feeling like a punching bag I resumed my regu-lar chiropractic adjustment with Paul. A few hours after each rotation chair session, I felt stiff and achy. Paul confirmed that my neck and back were out of alignment after almost every rotation therapy session. Although I was just sitting in the chair, the muscles in my neck, back, and shoulders were tightening to stabilize my balance. The balance system comprises your eyes, your ears, and your muscles. My muscles were getting a workout!

After attending a chair session to see how it worked, Paul decided to do cranial adjustments several times a week as well. Cranial work involves gentle pressure on my skull, including compression and stretching from various angles. Consistent with Colette's explanation, cranial adjustments disrupted the co-contractions. Almost immediately I was aware of less pres-sure in my head and ears after these sessions. The chiropractic manipula-tions and massages made it possible to continue the rotation therapy. Without this support I would not have been able to tolerate the aftereffects. I made sure Colette understood how essential this posttherapy therapy was when I talked to her about my symptoms.

In mid-August I was able to tolerate eight sets—a grand total of thirty-two minutes—with no symptoms. Because I was adapting in the therapy but not able to translate that adaptation to my real life, we decided to increase the velocity of the rotation. Whee! The dots rotating at greater speed increased the stimulus and made it harder to adapt. We started back at twelve minutes with this new program.

August 25, 2000

This week the effects of the new "high velocity" rotation therapy have held me down. It was quite overwhelming the first session—last Thursday. But I had five days to recover. This week I went Tuesday and Thursday and there went the week in a blur of nausea,

*unsteadiness and generally feeling a bit "off." The unusual thing
is that this week I have felt no impact during the therapy and no
real symptoms for the first two hours afterwards. Only then do I
begin to get nauseous, dizzy, headachy. On Tuesday I was awake all
night—the lights just kept rotating by my eyes and my brain was too
stimulated to allow me to sleep. Thankfully, I have all next week with
no therapy.*

This new pattern—the delayed reaction—matched my real-life experience. While I was in a crowd or on a drive, my symptoms weren't as severe
as they'd been in the past. Then, wham! Real symptoms emerged two to
four hours later. It thwarted my management strategy, because I planned to
leave an event when I felt symptoms. Now, if I stayed until I noticed symptoms, it was way too late. This explained a lot about why I'd gotten into
trouble at several recent events. I needed to change my strategy—to regu-
late my activities by the clock, not by the symptom.

Colette conferred further with Dr. Black about the change in my
symptom pattern. He immediately suggested I try a maneuver called a
hallpike. Hallpikes are done by sitting on a bed, with the head turned to
one side at a 45-degree angle and leaning back rapidly so your head is hanging off the side of the bed. When I had done this exercise in the past I often
felt dizzy or a sinking sensation for the first five to ten seconds my head
hung over the bed. Dr. Black instructed me to do hallpikes every night
before bed, repeating the maneuver with my head turned to each side, for
as many times as it took to remove all symptoms.

Then, my first hydrops episode of the year occurred, probably caused
by the summer heat and the increased stimulus of the faster rotation speed
during rotation chair sessions.

September 8, 2000

*Colette decided against my Tuesday therapy because I looked so
sick. It was silly to try to go. Once I was in the waiting room I could
tell I was in no shape for more stimulation—nauseous, shaky,
emotional—the fluorescent lights even bothered me. Colette did
speak to Dr. Black later in the day and he recommended a shift to
8 minutes at the fast speed—three times a week.*

*Last night Shelly was gone and I cried myself to sleep for the first
time in a long time. Just sad about limits, things that are in the past
that don't seem to be part of the future. And I prayed for help and
support—help to find the strength to explore the options, find the way.*

Who knows why these mini-crises arise—but then I had no illusion they would stop. They are a part of the process whether I understand the "why" of them or not.

This episode kept me isolated and resting for a few weeks. With the isolation came the opportunity to look back over the summer and try to understand what I learned. The Jewish New Year was approaching, so I was in rhythm with the larger need to reflect on my life and the direction I wanted for the next year.

My first obvious conclusions involved the therapy.

September 21, 2000

It seems that September is often a time of reflection and synthesis in my life—at least in this new limited life. I have to admit this summer has been difficult. Generally it took two days to recover after therapy and by that time I was due to go in again. With most sessions I was dizzy and shaky about an hour after and then got muscle aches, maybe a headache and nausea for the rest of the day. The next day I was only tired and unmotivated. Two days after I started to feel normal but was constipated from the effects on my digestive system. And then I headed back to start the cycle again. It is like a practicum in how to develop chronic fatigue. In these last few days I have had to face that I can't do the rehab as frequently—it is taking over my life, lowering my reserves—it is too much. The first step in the solution is simple—drop back to two times a week. The harder question is about whether this is working for me at all. Clearly I am adapting to the therapy but there are no significant leaps forward. . . . In the rest of my life the progress is barely noticeable. I don't know what I expected—actually that is a good sign, I don't think I expected anything. I wanted—I still want—to take all the steps I could to see if I could improve my condition—expand my limits.

I don't want to cling desperately to this therapy as my last chance, to keep pushing it regardless of results. On the other hand, I don't want to quit while I am still progressing. This is a mental bookmark to help me see if and when I become attached to continuing in the face of no progress. Not yet, but it is possible.

I started to feel so tired I felt flat, like in the days of chronic fatigue. I'd almost forgotten the feeling until I felt myself slipping back into the pit. I was not yet ready to stop trying, but I saw a limit to my ability to sustain my efforts.

After a week of rest and reflection, I resumed therapy. Colette started with two sets at the faster speed, but something had changed; I felt good and strong both at the session and afterwards. I was not sure whether the change was a result of the rest from the break in therapy or the hallpikes.

September 28, 2000

On the eve of the Jewish New Year, I am experiencing a breakthrough. At the very least the hallpikes I have been doing every night are totally eliminating the movement I felt when I was lying down to sleep. That has been true whether I was stirred up from the rotation chair or from the long drive to and from Bend. What that has meant is that I am really sleeping, I am refreshed by my sleep. So here only a week later than my last entry I can honestly say I am not as tired. I have been more energetic and motivated than any time I can recall with this illness. Even if the hallpikes were the only positive development, it would be enough. I am grateful for the ability to rest and recuperate. When you think about it, the recuperative powers of rest border on miraculous.

But there is more. In the past 10 days I have adapted to each new level of rotation—3 sets, 4 sets, 5 sets—with no symptoms. I am tired and I still get constipated for a day but there is no nausea, no dizziness, and no aching muscles. Clearly my brain is adapting to this new speed. It still remains to be seen whether or not I am adapting in my real life—can I go to synagogue, travel, go to events— even go out for dinner—without getting sick? This is new territory, there may be a possibility I can expand the boundaries, the fences around my life.

On the other hand, aside from feeling stronger overall, there is no evidence my crowd reaction has lessened. So I don't want to get ahead of myself. There is still the fact that the hallpikes stop the movement—consistently.

✳   ✳   ✳

The synagogue services for the High Holy Days provided an ideal testing ground for my new strength and energy. I stayed for two hours of services each of the first two days and on the third day stayed for more than one hour. Each day I was more tired than the day before and less able to tolerate the crowd motion. The first day—when I had no symptoms after two hours—I had the wild idea that I was going to be fine, no symptoms ever again! Once the delayed reaction set in I was forced to see I was a little stronger and slightly better able to tolerate the motion, but this was not a dramatic breakthrough. Every individual has a slightly different pattern of motion that triggers vestibular symptoms. The motion pattern in the synagogue clearly was my trigger.

October 1, 2000

Oddly enough, even after getting my hopes up, I am not disappointed. I've spent almost 5 years now taking one small, slow step after the other. While I pray that I will be able to travel, to go to lectures, to attend synagogue, I no longer feel desperate or hard edged. I think I can do those things now, with care and rest, with awareness. I don't resent the need for awareness. So if I can continue to make some progress, just a little more, and maybe a little more. I have tried as hard and persevered as long as I know how. I am certain that I have not been poor in spirit. I feel I have endured and I have been greatly rewarded.

October 4, 2000

I am finding I am not discouraged by the lack of therapy breakthroughs translating into real life breakthroughs. I was not sure how I was going to react when this option was finished. I can see now I did not expect it to change things. There is no sense of failure or giving up, there is acceptance. I will still fight against limits at times, I don't expect to graciously accept everything about this forever. But somewhere inside I had concluded the changes were fundamental— and their effects were probably permanent. I don't recall if I have ever let go so completely of future progress in healing—but I think this is new. I will do those things I can do, I will try new things and try to increase my tolerance to crowds—but life as I knew it is over. It won't ever be the same again. Even if I am very successful at further progress, the best I see is visits to that life—not permanent residency. The depth of the acceptance is reflected in my inability to feel either sad or unmoved. It is just what it is.

October 2, 2000

I was walking with Bunkee along Balch Creek after a torrential downpour all night. The creek was a muddy river after all the runoff and leaves were falling. At one point I looked up and saw a leaf just as it began a graceful, swinging descent into the creek. It was so gentle, so soft and slow. For the past several years I have been reminded of the cycle of life and death so strongly by the leaves in the fall. This particular leaf recalled my father's gentle, fading death. It would seem to indicate a special life to deserve such a peaceful and graceful death. Later in the day I was watching TV as I ate dinner—Shelly is gone—and caught a moment of a nature show filming an elephant grieving for her dead calf. She and the herd had returned to the spot where its skull and parts of the skeleton still lay. She touched the bones, encircled them with her trunk, and probed all the openings—making low keening sounds. It was as moving a picture of grief as I have ever seen. Both these images reminded me strongly of how deeply I miss my father. There is a permanent ache in my heart, a piece missing, a piece of my love that calls out and can't be answered. I am at peace with the grief and the loss—which means I don't struggle with it, not that I don't feel it.

I was finishing three years of treatment (after a year and a half seeking a diagnosis) with no additional treatments or therapies on the immediate horizon. The conclusion of the final therapy—the long-awaited rotation chair—left me with no dramatic improvement and no further options. I realized I was entering the final stage of healing: acceptance.

Speaking From Experience: Tips to Make Your Journey Easier

1. I never consciously tried to reach a point of acceptance of my vestibular disorders but, once there, I recognized a fundamental shift. In order for my new life to begin, my old life needed to reach closure. I had to accept my new direction, my new life. Acceptance was a significant emotional milestone, even more important than the practical milestone of beginning to manage my own medical team. I was no longer torn between looking back at my past life and looking forward to an unknown future. I was no longer suspended in limbo. I began to look forward with a sense of clarity and, perhaps, adventure!

2. One of the most beneficial supportive therapies for me was chiropractic work. I was fortunate to have a chiropractor who was interested in my specific illness. He even visited a rotation therapy appointment to understand the fundamental challenge causing my need for adjustment. Without this understanding, he might not have started the cranial manipulation that was so beneficial to me. It was useful to describe my vestibular disorders to my other medical doctors so they were better able understand my needs and anticipate problems.

3. A delayed reaction to vestibular challenges is not uncommon, but it is tricky to manage. I started by experimenting with exposure times. I tried staying in a crowd for an hour, left, and observed whether or not I had symptoms. If I did, I cut back on the time. If I didn't, I increased the time. Fairly soon, I was able to decide not only what I could do, or what I was willing to try, but also for how long.

4. After all my experiments with driving and symptoms after long drives, I drew one clear conclusion for me: The car matters. My symptoms were significantly less when the car was higher and quieter and the ride was smoother. Other factors, like windshield wipers moving and approaching headlights, exacerbated symptoms, but those are common to all cars. One summer Shelly and I rented every model of SUV to see which car was best for me before we bought a new car.

18

Testing Acceptance

NOVEMBER 2000–SEPTEMBER 2002

December 18, 2000

I can choose to try new therapies, I can do the exercises, I can rest enough, etc. And I can also choose the level of activity I engage in—I can choose my challenges. With all these tools I build a life and I can feel well—under limits, most of the time. Or, I can be more active and feel less well. It sounds obvious but I had not really seen it quite so clearly. The illness is both my reactions to the motion as it is the resultant controlled life I must choose to feel well.

December 25, 2000

I can't put a value on the closure and clarity the writing has provided in my healing. As I re-read and rewrite it is almost as if this happened to someone else. Without the aid of daily writing, recording of symptoms—but even more without trying to pull it all together and make sense of it, I could not have seen the depth of meaning and reached a peace with it all.

For most of 2001 my symptoms were relatively stable. I continued to experience motion sickness in crowds. I experimented with various strategies, including medications, exposure times, noise impact and exercises after the crowd exposure. I also observed symptoms after every drive to our vacation house in central Oregon and after every flight. For days afterward I felt like I was moving, even when I was lying down. I also felt dizzy, unable to think clearly or speak, and I was nauseous. The odd thing was that I never felt bad while I was traveling. I thought this was *mal de debarquement*, but I had no idea what to do to prevent or lessen the symptoms. Despite these recurring problems, I felt consistently better in 2001. There were no significant new problems, and my life expanded ever so slightly.

These observations and conclusions about the healing process were tested in late 2001 when I suddenly began to experience persistent vertigo. In 1996, when I first got sick, I experienced vertigo, but it dissipated after a few weeks and recurred infrequently. I'd had one similar episode in 1999, but this continual vertigo was my first new symptom in years. After a few weeks it settled into a pattern of dramatic spinning whenever I turned my head to the right while lying down. I waited a few weeks before making an appointment with Dr. Black because symptoms frequently resolved or changed. I wanted to have a better perspective and more observations to share.

It took Dr. Black only a few minutes to diagnose *benign paroxysmal positional nystagmus* (BPPN), which occurs when extremely small crystals, called *otoliths*, dislodge from their usual location and get stuck in another part of the inner ear. There are three possible ear canals the little crystals could rest in to cause vertigo. When one of these crystals lodged in an ear canal my gyroscope went "Tilt!" As the otoliths moved around in my ear I felt like I was spinning or the room was spinning.

> Benign paroxysmal positional nystagmus, or BPPN, occurs when extremely small crystals, called otoliths, dislodge from their usual location and get stuck in another part of the inner ear.

Within minutes I was in the treatment room with Colette. She put a pair of bulky goggles on my eyes that had tiny video cameras filming my eye movement and transmitting that video to a computer screen. As I did hallpikes my eyes moved involuntarily, and Colette watched these movements on the screen. The hallpikes stir up the crystals so the BPPN is evident, both to the patient and to the doctor. When Colette ran the video for Dr. Black it confirmed his diagnosis—my eyes jumped wildly when I experienced vertigo. These wild eye movements have a medical name: *nystagmus*.

> The treatment for BPPN is called canalith repositioning procedure (CRP).

The treatment for BPPN is called *canalith repositioning procedure* (CRP), and it began immediately. On the basis of the eye movements Dr. Black could identify which ear canal the loose particles were in. Dr. Black and Colette turned me in various positions—basically a 360-degree rotation while lying down on an exam table—and observed the changes to my eye movements. A rapidly vibrating device was placed around my ear to shake the particles out of their current, irritating location. Dr. Black could tell when the particles moved by tracking my eye movement. It was very interesting but not immediately effective. Dr. Black reassured me it often took several CRP sessions to clear up the problem.

After the treatment I sat in the waiting room for half an hour to let the vertigo subside so I could drive home. The effects of strong vertigo often lingered for hours, and I felt very dizzy, off balance, and nauseous. For forty-eight hours after each CRP session I had to keep my head upright. This kept the otoliths from falling back into the wrong place and allowed them to reabsorb. I became very adept at bending my knees rather than my neck to do things like retrieve items from low cabinets, brush my teeth, or wash dishes. I never did become adept at sleeping with my head elevated, but I did it.

The episodes were unwelcome, but at least BPPN was a vestibular problem with a clear diagnosis and an effective treatment. CRP was very effective for most patients—more than ninety percent were cured with one or two treatments. Plus, the vertigo was position specific—I experienced it only when my head moved into certain positions. If I avoided those positions I was fairly successful at avoiding the vertigo. I learned that lying or sleeping on my right side was not a good idea. I also quickly learned that looking up and to the right was ill advised. I could try to disperse the crystals by performing the hallpike maneuver at home. My initial reaction to adding BPPN to my list of vestibular problems was muted by a false sense of control.

In the latter part of 2001, hydrops episodes began to recur and sometimes lasted for as long as three to four months, becoming intertwined with the BPPN episodes. The hydrops exacerbated the vertigo from BPPN, and the BPPN in turn exacerbated the constant dizziness and nausea from the hydrops. Also, any crowd motion or travel made it all just that much worse.

For almost nine months starting in the summer of 2001 I struggled with almost constant severe symptoms. My early optimism about the BPPN diagnosis and treatment faded. To make matters worse, the CRP, so effective in treating BPPN for others, did not appear to be very effective for me. Acceptance faded away.

Throughout the revolving hydrops and BPPN episodes I saw Dr. Black for various tests. We tried new diuretics for the hydrops, blood tests to check for potassium and other deficiencies, and an MRI and a computerized tomography scan to assess whether there was another reason for the vertigo. Dr. Black suspected a semicircular canal dehiscence (absence of enough bone around the ear canal.) It was important to rule out that possibility with the computerized tomography scans and MRI. Like many times before, the symptoms of this problem were similar but the root cause was different, and we needed to treat the root cause. As Dr. Black was fond of saying, "This would all be easier if we could just lift up the hood and look at it."

My third BPPN episode, in February 2002, stubbornly failed to resolve with the traditional CRP. Dr. Black consulted a colleague, Dr. John Epley, also located in Portland. Dr. Epley did pioneering work in diagnosing and treating BPPN. He had invented a device that allowed him to position a patient at any angle in space to better locate the crystals in the various ear canals (there are three) and therefore make more precise adjustments. The device was potentially effective but as patient friendly as a pit bull. Imagine hanging upside down, blindfolded and strapped to a chair while all the professionals, with their backs to the patient, view your filmed eye movements in a corner of the room on a computer screen. It was not exactly torture, but close. (Shelly said he kept thinking of the Spanish Inquisition as he watched the procedure.) As they spoke medical jargon in hushed tones, it was a great comfort to know that Shelly was there also—eyes on me.

This treatment approach was no more effective for me than the CRPs, and it caused worse symptoms. Shelly and I decided that enough was enough. For now, tolerating the vertigo was more acceptable than additional treatment.

On the basis of my experience and Dr. Black's calm explanations, I understood that when several vestibular problems are present at the same time it is more challenging to untangle them and arrive at a solution. As the untangling proceeded I turned my focus to sleep difficulties.

I had begun to experience insomnia. Each night I fell asleep immediately only to wake up two or three hours later and remain awake for hours. If I was lucky, I would fall asleep again for a few hours in the early morning. Lack of sleep on top of dizziness and balance issues was intolerable.

April 29, 2002

I'm losing track of why I even care what is wrong at this point. I'm uncertain of my ability to distinguish a normal day from a bad day. I don't know if I have just forgotten how it feels not to be dizzy and exhausted or if I am imagining I feel dizzier and more exhausted than other people. I've felt depressed for a few days—astoundingly a few gorgeous, sunny days. Nothing serious but on the verge of tears and sad. It would make sense that I am just worn out from sleeping less than 5 hours a night for 6 months. But who knows.

Dr. Black referred me to a local sleep expert for testing. Rest is critical to recuperate from the effects of balance disorders. An underlying sleep disorder, which many balance patients have, has to be treated in order to make vestibular progress.

Rest is critical to recuperate from the effects of balance disorders. An underlying sleep disorder, which many balance patients have, has to be treated in order to make vestibular progress.

The sleep clinic was another fascinating adventure. The objective was to identify a physical cause of my disturbed sleep pattern. I had my usual performance anxiety, afraid this would be the first night in months I would sleep straight through! I was wired up with electrodes, ushered to a lovely stage set of a bedroom, and plugged in. There was an attendant in an adjoining room who watched my brain waves and monitored whether or not the equipment was working and I was okay. This was the very embodiment of Big Brother watching over me.

I experienced my typical pattern. I woke up and knew I couldn't go back to sleep, so I decided to go ahead and meditate like I always did because it gives me some needed relaxation. When I stopped meditating the attendant came in to see how I was doing and ask if I was meditating—the brain pattern on the electrodes gave me away.

The doctor came in early to review the data and talk with each of the three sleepers who were in the sleep clinic that night. In my case he said he wished he could have gotten more data—meaning he wished I'd slept a bit longer. That made two of us! On the basis of what he saw, there was no physical reason, other than my vestibular problems, for my lack of sleep. This was the result I had expected.

The sleep doctor described several medications to help me sleep but wanted to confer with Dr. Black before making a final recommendation. Dr. Black ruled out all of his recommendations because those specific medications exacerbated balance problems. I pointed out that my antinausea medication, Phenergan, made me drowsy and that I slept well when I used it for nausea. Dr. Black was satisfied that using Phenergan as a sleep aid would not exacerbate my balance problems.

At the same time, my other test results ruled out other complications and I was left with a diagnosis of fluctuating hydrops and BPPN. In the spirit of solving one problem at a time, I resolved to stabilize my sleep and see what benefits accrued for the other problems. I devised an eight-week recovery plan of reduced activity and increased sleep—using Phenergan—and rest to see if I could regain equilibrium. If I did not feel better after eight weeks, I vowed to explore additional steps. What those would be I did not know.

A large part of my life focused on the continuing symptoms and the cycle of activity, sickness, and recovery, but I was also trying to live a fairly normal life. Shelly and I drove the more than three hours to our wonderful house on the Deschutes River every three to four weeks. Our time there was magical, an island of calm and quiet filled with birds, mountains, and seemingly endless walks through wilderness forests. There was no denying my symptoms after the drives—I began to see that the drive coming back was noticeably harder than the drive going over—but the time spent there between drives was rejuvenating.

We also maintained our schedule of twice-yearly family visits to Los Angeles and North Carolina. Staying close to our families was a priority for both of us. My mother had completely recovered from her broken hip and wrist and was more active than ever. We even met my sister Jill and her family in Vancouver, British Columbia, when they were heading up to Whistler for a skiing vacation. Vancouver has always been one of our favorite cities, and the opportunity to visit again with family was irresistible. The five-hour drive was more than I could tolerate, and recovery took more than a week, but I knew that when I agreed to go.

The new element in my daily life was the synagogue remodel. During the past three years, Shelly and I had worked together leading a large committee through the fund raising and then renovation design phases. All the meetings with the congregation to gather input on the design were over, and construction began. Shelly was working as hard as ever, so I was the person who hopped into the car and went to the synagogue on a moment's notice to deal with daily construction issues. I also ordered all the furniture and was responsible for approving the items as they arrived. Synagogue members walked through the building daily to check on the status of their synagogue, so there were always issues. This project took two to three hours a day, which was as close to all consuming as I could tolerate. Other things, like writing and painting, fell to the side.

Moments of feeling aimless and useless were a thing of the past.

May 10, 2002

I've been running around like an idiot these past few days. Yesterday, the synagogue construction and today, just the business of life. There are only three more weeks before the remodel is finished and it is coming together rapidly and beautifully. There are the usual hassles, complaints, frantic decisions . . . but overall it is everything we envisioned and more. I guess I was running on vapors because I feel awful today.

What was not a thing of the past was my inability to monitor how I was feeling and to set my schedule to maintain my energy and health. I was still rising to occasions and suffering the aftereffects, but there are some projects and activities that set their own schedule and are worthwhile despite the impact. The symptoms are temporary, whereas the results are more long lasting.

May 30, 2002

Yesterday I put into words what Shelly and I have been focused on with our work at the synagogue over the past year. I saw the difficulty of handing down a tradition from generation to generation. Specifically the difficulty of the older generation making a handoff, and the younger group accepting the handoff and moving forward confidently. While there are endless hassles, confusions and panics, when I step back I can see the meaning. Shelly and I have been a part of accepting the baton, of being a strong link in the chain, of gaining the confidence of our elders and our peers and delivering a result that I hope will delight them. There is great meaning and reward in forging our own link in the chain.

In August 2002, the new sanctuary was dedicated, with a ribbon cutting and a Torah processional around the block. The synagogue was filled with proud, happy members celebrating a renewal of our religious home.

At the dedication banquet I sat next to an Israeli woman, Gillie, who was currently living in Portland. We chatted politely, and each of us mentioned that the banquet setting was difficult because we had some health problems. I was avoiding the inevitable mention of vestibular problems that no one had ever heard of. I was astounded to find that Gillie was also a vestibular patient of Dr. Black's. My first vestibular friend! Neither of us spoke to anyone else at the table all evening! It was so exciting, so gratifying to find someone who understood our secret language of dizziness and balance.

Gillie's balance story was far more dramatic than mine. When she and her youngest daughter were in Spain they were hit by a bus and dragged under it. After six months in a coma and healing from her obvious injuries for more than a year, Gillie met Dr. Black while seeking help for her daughter's continuing balance and dizziness symptoms. Dr. Black referred Gillie's daughter to a pediatric specialist. Their conversation, however, helped Gillie realize she had balance problems as well—perilymph fistulas. Gillie's fistulas were caused by the catastrophic impact of her collision with the bus. She was struggling with symptoms very similar to mine, but she was earlier in the discovery process. She still believed this was a problem that would resolve with treatment.

To compound Gillie's predicament, she had two young daughters, and her husband had left her about a year earlier. She was a single parent, without a U.S. work permit, trying to support two daughters while she experienced continued dizziness, nausea, headaches, and fatigue. She was also highly educated (she had a PhD in international marketing) and motivated professional who was deeply frustrated by her inability to work. I was excited to have a friend who shared parts of my experience but humbled by Gillie's challenges and hesitant to dampen her optimism and determination with my story. We started to walk together every week, growing closer and closer.

✳   ✳   ✳

Shelly and I planned to go to Scotland in September to meet up with my sister Anne and her partner, Matt. This was our first major vacation outside the normal routine of family visits and weekends in Bend in several years.

Shelly and I went to Edinburgh and Glasgow by ourselves, then joined Anne and Matt for hiking in the Highlands. This first week on our own allowed me to get over my dizziness, nausea, and sleeplessness from the long airplane trip. It also provided a wonderful opportunity for Shelly and me to rediscover how much we liked to travel together. We weren't much for the big tourist sites. We liked to pretend we lived in the place—take long walks, explore the local gardens and architecture, linger in cafes, and shop in the local grocery stores. We even attended Rosh Hashanah services in the old Garnet Hill synagogue in Glasgow.

The second week, the four of us stayed in a remote railway cottage in the Highlands and tramped through rough country and rocky paths. It was dramatically beautiful—misty and rugged, and Matt was an intrepid leader. I felt well enough to do most of the group hikes and events. We were in Urquhart Castle on September 11 when the PA system came on and asked everyone to observe a minute of silence on the solemn anniversary of the attacks on the World Trade Center and the Pentagon. I was struck by the respect and introspection of every person around me. It was especially meaningful to be outside the United States remembering and honoring the memory.

I also found some new—or undiscovered—limitations.

September 25, 2002

Along the way I discovered urban train rides with structures flashing by the window cause symptoms. I was very dismayed to find I could not hike on rocky paths where I needed to balance each foot at every step—it made me too dizzy and I started to spin and lose balance. After ¼ mile I was forced to turn back. Anne and Matt were very understanding and Shelly was fabulous. Shelly and I headed back for an 8 mile walk along the lovely country road to Glen Nevis. We truly enjoyed ambling along at our own pace enjoying the scenery.

All in all, it was a good trip. Shelly and I were able to get away from the pressures and responsibilities of his work. I was encouraged by my flexibility—my graceful acceptance—of the new limits. There was no emotional reaction, simply a readjustment.

We arrived home to celebrate the remainder of Jewish High Holy Days with the accompanying religious as well as social festivities—and the usual dizziness, nausea, and spinning. Shelly and I invited my new dizzy friend, Gillie, to dinner as a part of the holiday celebration.

September 27, 2002

Gillie said she had a wonderful time at our house for dinner but it was also depressing—because of how limited my life is—much more than she had hoped. And she saw that she hadn't accepted that for herself, so it was depressing. Although I don't have any real insight about whether or not she will get 100% better, experience tells me the chances are slim. Experience also tells me she needs to find out for herself. I told her we had different conditions and people even seem to respond differently to the same condition—so she needed to focus on her own healing and not assume she'd have my same limits. She thanked me for that reassurance with full awareness—and I truly hope she can find a wider range of activity.

Speaking From Experience: Tips to Make Your Journey Easier

1. Setbacks presented difficult emotional and physical challenges. I knew the healing would not be linear, that I would reach plateaus and that there would be setbacks. Understanding these things intellectually and tolerating the setback with patience and grace were two different things entirely. This particular setback lasted more than a year, compounded

by new problems. All I could do was what I knew: consult Dr. Black, stick to his advice as closely as possible, plan fewer and shorter activities, and try to find the patience to endure without losing hope.

2. One part of enduring without losing hope was gaining a sense of progress with the vestibular problem of the moment. With multiple problems it is essential to peel problems away one by one. The first success was the insomnia; Phenergan has reliably helped me sleep in my dizziest of times. This was critical because rest and recovery are so central to vestibular healing. I was unsuccessful at eliminating the BPPN, but I was able to tolerate it by avoiding the head position that caused the strongest vertigo. I had to satisfy my self with progress on these two fronts as Dr. Black and I worked hard to identify the root cause of the cycling hydrops.

3. I want to say just a word about friends with vestibular disorders. I felt very isolated and lonely with vestibular problems and not only because I was alone quite a lot. I had never read about anyone else with vestibular problems, no one I spoke with had ever heard of vestibular problems, and I certainly didn't know anyone else with vestibular problems. When I met Gillie, the connection was strong and immediate despite our very different circumstances. We struggled with the same hopes and fears—the same symptoms and the same desires to get well. We understood each other without explanation. Neither of us tended to complain. Instead, we compared notes on symptoms: what were mine or hers, how did we each manage them, were they getting better? We explored our otherwise-unspoken concerns about our futures, and we laughed a lot. There are numerous vestibular support groups listed on www.vestibular.org, including face-to-face as well as online groups. Perhaps your doctor could also help you connect with another patient with vestibular disorders.

19

A Genuine Breakthrough

OCTOBER 2002–OCTOBER 2003

After a very pleasant dinner at Gillie's one October night, I felt ear pressure and dizziness on the way home. I took Phenergan so I could sleep, because I continued to feel movement inside as well as outside my head. I assumed this was my normal reaction to crowds; there had been nine of us at dinner. I woke up at 4:00 a.m. very dizzy and reeled when I tried to walk. I suspected benign paroxysmal positional nystagmus (BPPN), so I checked to see what happened when I lay flat on my back with my head slightly turned to the right. Bingo! The room whirled wildly.

I was still in a revolving BPPN and hydrops cycle, so I took a few days to prepare a summary of my symptoms as well as my activity on both good and bad days before seeing Dr. Black. Just to be certain I was communicating clearly I also provided definitions of all the symptoms, including reeling; vertigo; and feeling shaky, dizzy, off balance. Finally, I listed a series of specific situations that caused severe or unusual symptoms.

Dr. Black's zest for research kicked into high gear with all these data. He confirmed my suspicions about BPPN. In addition, he suspected I had an ongoing active hydrops episode. He pointed out that my persistent nausea and in particular my severe symptoms after flights could indicate a reopened fistula. Reopened fistulas—*my worst fear!* There was no benefit to leaping off that bridge yet, however. First things first.

I scheduled an electrocochleography test to confirm hydrops. The test showed that my hydrops was severely out of control despite my regular diuretic and hydrating regimen. Getting this hydrops under control was my highest priority. I refused to think about a reopened fistula. That would mean another long bed rest and year of recovery and no activity—too daunting.

After the electrocochleography test results, the discussion with Dr. Black focused on my diet. I mentioned that I was a vegetarian and had been for almost thirty years but that over the past few years I had added a small amount of fish to my diet. To my shock and dismay, he explained that a vegetarian diet could be viewed as a major cause of the hydrops and that it was unlikely I was getting enough protein. Vestibular professionals were just beginning to understand a connection between a Zone-type diet and treatment of hydrops. The Zone Diet is a specifically prescribed balance of protein, carbohydrates, and fat consumed in multiple small meals over the day. In addition to other benefits, the Zone Diet promotes a stable fluid balance essential to hydrops prevention. I was skeptical.

> To my shock and dismay, Dr. Black explained that a vegetarian diet could be viewed as a major cause of the hydrops and that it was unlikely I was getting enough protein.

Dr. Black was convinced that my vegetarian diet was the root cause of these persistent, recurring episodes that defied the usual diuretic control. I was not convinced, but I started on the Zone Diet at his recommendation. Once I reviewed the diet, I could see that my vegetarian diet was indeed woefully deficient in protein. I continued to eat primarily a vegetarian diet, relying on soy protein, but I also added more fish. The results were rapid and positive: I began to feel less nauseated and experienced far less dizziness within a week.

November 19, 2002

When I saw Fran from Dr. Black's office a week ago I had already made one step of improvement with just 6 days on the diet—the vertigo was gone and the pressure had diminished slightly in my ears. Today I feel I stepped up another notch—the pressure has been diminishing steadily—all of a sudden the world looks clearer and crisper. I felt I could see better, there was no fog or blur. So I know I am improving, all I can ask for.

Adjusting to the new diet was challenging. I became that person who reads every label. It wasn't just a matter of whether or not yogurt, for example, conformed to the diet. It was necessary to find THE yogurt that provided the closest acceptable balance of protein, carbs, and fat according to Zone recommendations. This made for long grocery trips!

As with any new diet, meal planning and eating in restaurants was difficult for the first month until I got the hang of how strict I needed to be and cemented my understanding of what was primarily protein or carbohydrate or fat. Many foods—dairy, for example—contained some of each, to varying degrees, depending on the particular product.

By December it was clear to me, and to Dr. Black, that the majority of my severe symptoms were going away as my "out of control" hydrops went away. When I reported no vertigo, less dizziness and nausea, greatly decreased ear pressure, and improved energy, we were both smiling from ear to ear. The diet was working! The longer I stayed on this diet, and the more closely I followed it, the better I felt. My hydrops episodes were shorter and less frequent.

This was a huge positive development—huge! Hydrops episodes were a constant part of my life. I had two to three debilitating episodes a year, each one lasting months. They magnified all the other dizziness and out-of-balance symptoms I tried to manage every day. They were also confusing. The symptoms came on slowly and were hard to identify because there was so much overlap with other problems, like fistulas and BPPN. I felt so powerful and so happy to have the Zone Diet as a tool!

The scientific background readings on the Zone Diet also addressed the biochemical effects of stress on the body. Conflicting balance signals put my body under constant stress. When I added emotional stress, or more demanding balance challenges, significant physical responses were entirely predictable: I overloaded my stress quotient. I loved it when I found explanations for what I experienced, and here was the explanation for my diminished ability to tolerate stress.

In addition to resolving the hydrops, the diet success assuaged my fear of reopened fistulas. I wouldn't be losing a year to bed rest and recovery! More immediately, this meant I would be able to make my planned speech to the American Association of Otolaryngology.

While Shelly and I were in Scotland, I received a request from Dr. Black to speak on a panel during the annual meeting of the Association for Research in Otolaryngology (ARO) in Florida in February 2003. He was working with the Vestibular Disorders Association, to develop a roster of speakers to illustrate the experience of vestibular illness from a patient's perspective. I was committed to working for greater awareness and understanding of vestibular problems, so this was a golden opportunity.

December 16, 2002

Dr. Black is pleased at the results of the diet and excited about the Florida meeting. He's at a point in his career where he has something to say that he feels strongly about, where he needs the attention of his colleagues. He is concerned about the low levels of research into vestibular illness and the low entry rate of new doctors. I hope I can live up to his expectations. In my heart I am confident that I am supposed to do this and that I have all the skills I need to do it as well as anyone. Just the opportunity gives meaning to these long years of trying to figure it out.

*   *   *

My list of vestibular problems and complications was shrinking for the first time in years. Yes, the motion sickness in crowds and the travel symptoms from *mal de debarquement* were still there, as was the BPPN, but I had powerful tools to manage both the hydrops and the insomnia. I realized I was going to have my typical ups and downs—for example, after driving to Bend or visiting family. I hoped the downs would not be as dramatic as they had been over the past few years. Without the fog of the constant hydrops, I could also see my role in the cycles more clearly.

January 28, 2003

It's not that any of this is new, it's that it isn't. This is it. This is my life. Feeling pretty lousy most of the time with moments, hours . . . and hopefully days . . . when I am able to forget it. Perhaps part of the reason I like to feel busy is to escape focusing on it. But I still need to fine tune my ability to strike a balance. I'm making choices to do certain things and not others fairly well. And I need to bring that sense of choice and balance more actively into every day—not just outside events.

I began to plan my speech to the ARO. The meeting was now less than a month away. I received a draft of the workshop plan and was interested to read about the theme:

ARO members are developing new genetic and cellular therapeutic mechanisms for diagnosing and rehabilitating hearing loss. For decades there have been standard diagnostic tools to determine the degree of hearing loss, its cause and its epidemiology and extent in society. Yet this is manifestly not the case with vestibular disorders. Vestibular disorders are typically misdiagnosed and are often treated with clinical indifference or misunderstanding leading to poor data required for epidemiological studies.

It was maddening, sad, frustrating, and very, very disappointing to read this confirmation from the professional community even though it reflected my experience. My role at the seminar was to illustrate—first hand—the impact of vestibular disorders on an individual's life. Other panelists were professionals in the field who would be addressing the epidemiology of vestibular disorders and highlighting the problems facing vestibular researchers. As I understood it, we were all in sales, hoping to entice researchers to enter the vestibular field. This was no small responsibility, even though I had no illusions about how much a short speech can really hope to accomplish.

In early February, I started making the speech to Bunkee and Looey. They loved it! A few days before the departure I got a case of pretrip jitters. I realized I had never even considered the stress of the trip and the speech. I had agreed to give the speech because I thought it was important to increase awareness of vestibular illness. I had never thought about the vestibular downside of the stress, the long airplane trip, and the number of people at the meeting—certainly large enough to constitute a crowd.

Shelly and I planned the trip to allow some recovery time before my speech, so we were in Daytona Beach a few days early. It was chilly and overcast, not to mention more than a little dingy, which made it easy to spend most of the time in our room, resting. I was dizzy and off balance, still vibrating from the flight and dealing with my typical posttrip nausea. We took a few long walks every day, but nothing seemed to help very much. The stress of the upcoming performance was adding to my other physical challenges. Although I had given dozens of speeches each year for the past two decades, there was no denying it: I was nervous!

March 7, 2003

Oddly enough, once I walked into the room—a huge ballroom set up for about 600 people—I was fine. I figure there were 150 people there and I was able to do the presentation as always—being myself, making eye contact, speaking from my heart. The preparation with Bunkee and Looey paid off. I must say I enjoyed the old familiar sense of command, the performance. I don't miss it and I wouldn't sacrifice to have it again—but it's a pleasure to feel competent.

Shelly and I also listened to Dr. Black and the [National Institutes of Health] presentation which were really interesting.

I thought the speech had gone well, and Dr. Black was very pleased with his colleagues' response to my remarks. That alone made the whole trip worthwhile.

Now that the nerve-wracking part was over, Shelly and I headed for stage two of the Florida trip: a relaxing time in the Florida Keys. It was warm and sunny and featured miles of turquoise water. It was probably all the beautiful water that lured me onto a boat—or that made me lure Shelly onto a small boat, despite previous warnings. I just wanted to try it for a short while, to do a little snorkeling. The trip was going fine until we slipped into the water to snorkel and found nothing but fifteen feet of murky water. Then we started the short trip back to shore and were rapidly overtaken by a huge cabin cruiser on autopilot. The wake from the cabin cruiser swamped our little boat and nearly sank it. Once we knew we were going to stay afloat it was hilarious—except for the fact that our cell phone and binoculars died from the salt water.

This short excursion confirmed that the original warnings against boating were more than justified. I had no symptoms when I was on the boat, but within hours they dizziness, nausea, and headache started. My intestinal tract locked up completely, and I was up all night with very painful constipation and stomach cramps. I spent most of my time pacing around the room, telling myself how stupid it had been to test my ability to handle a short boat ride. Sometimes I just needed to live, to have normal experiences and disregard the limits in order to have a life. This was not one of those times; this was stupid.

When we got home I called Dr. Black's nurse, Fran, to ask her about trying meclizine for my crowd and motion symptoms. She and Dr. Black had suggested it several times as a medication that sometimes helps and sometimes doesn't but was worth a try. I was in one of those stages where I wanted to try everything available because I'd just been through an experience that tested my limits. I quickly learned that meclizine didn't work for me.

Fran also told me Dr. Black was very pleased with the speech and the questions he received from colleagues afterward. I was happy he felt good about it.

The speech was a catalyst for me on other fronts as well. When I prepared my remarks for the ARO meeting, I relied heavily on my symptom tracking and notes of doctors' appointments. The data I had compiled and the conclusions and insights I had recorded were instrumental in giving me the confidence to speak. It reinforced my sense that I had something important to say. If anything, attendance at the ARO meeting increased my desire to make some contribution to a greater recognition and understanding of vestibular illness.

✳   ✳   ✳

After a trip to North Carolina in late April, I started to experience vertigo in addition to my usual postflight symptoms. Dr. Black hypothesized that, given my odd collection of symptoms, the vertigo could be due to protein deposits from severe hydrops rather than otoliths from BPPN. I asked about treatment for protein deposits, and Dr. Black described an approach that destroys ear function. When the ear's balance function is so haywire it hurts rather than helps the best treatment option is to remove the signals from the ear and let the eyes and muscles do the job of sending signals to the brain. Dr. Black also described a list of accompanying risks.

Given this frightening option, I was eager for another appointment with Dr. John Epley and the privilege of hanging upside down in his chair. The chair was very useful this time. The group of doctors was able to identify otoliths in both the posterior canal and the horizontal canal. Of the three possible ear canals in which the little crystals could rest to cause vertigo, they were dispersed in at least two of mine. This was a clear indicator that the culprit was BPPN.

June 16, 2003

Here's the story: my vertigo keeps returning so I must have periodic showering of otoliths. Frequently my nystagmus/vertigo is not strong which indicates dispersion of the crystals. Once they are dispersed the CPR—canalith repositioning—is less likely to work. Given all this, I can either live with the vertigo or have a risky surgery. Right now I choose to live with the vertigo.

The surgical solution to BPPN involves plugging the ear canal so that the otoliths could not enter and cause vertigo. Dr. Black explained that one of the risks of the surgery was the possibility of exacerbating my hydrops. I might have viewed that trade-off differently if I had not just met Kay, my second vestibular friend.

> The surgical solution to BPPN involves plugging the ear canal so that the otoliths cannot enter and cause vertigo.

Kay was from San Jose, California, and another patient of Dr. Black's. Fran had called me and described Kay's situation. She was coming to live in Portland for four to five months for treatment of her vestibular problems. She didn't have any other connection to Portland. Fran asked me to call her and meet her. When I called Kay it was awkward for both of us. We were both judicious with our time and attendance at social gatherings because of the balance problems. Plus, we were both independent and choosy about our friendships. I met her one morning at her hotel for breakfast, and we were fast friends from the moment I asked if we could eat on the deserted outside patio—in the 50-degree drizzle—to avoid the crowd in the break-fast room. Kay broke into a huge smile as she pulled on her raincoat.

Kay's overall situation was similar to mine. She was my age, married with no children, and she had a successful professional career editing and publishing nursing journals as well as providing nurses' training. She was also a former athlete—a swimmer, skier, and surfer. Her health challenges started with thyroid issues, and for the past several years she had struggled to find diagnosis and treatment for her balance problems. With all the medical resources at her disposal, she had chosen Dr. Black and made the commitment to live temporarily in Portland in order to receive treatment from him.

Kay had severe hydrops episodes every two weeks. The dizziness was so debilitating that she walked with a cane and was unable to walk very far because the motion of the wind in the trees or of passersby unsettled her. Yes, wind blowing in the trees made her dizzy! She was unable to read for more than a few minutes or watch TV—the movement and flicker of the screen triggered her symptoms. Yet there was absolutely nothing pathetic about Kay; she was smart, pragmatic, funny, and tough. She was also a keen observer of her symptoms and the situations that triggered them. When we were together we compared notes on vestibular oddities like this one:

Did that "Stop" sign just move when you looked up at it?

Yes, it did!

How far did it move?

Let me think . . . I'd say about six inches.

Hmmm . . . same for me. Isn't that interesting?

At this point we collapsed into giggles at how wonderful it was to have a friend for whom the signs also moved—and moved the same amount.

Kay was my shining example of "worse" hydrops, and I didn't want to invite those additional challenges. There were some crowd situations in which she was far less affected than I, and in those situations she took care of me. But I cherished my reading and walking and gardening. There would be no surgery for me; I would live with the vertigo.

Life perked along. I spent a great deal of time recovering from various events, but they were the kind of events that give joy and meaning to life—time with family and good friends. I relied on Paul, my trusty chiropractor, to help me recover more rapidly. He was becoming an expert in treating vestibular problems and was routinely using cranial-sacral manipulation in our sessions with promising results. The very gentle pressure from the manipulation of my skull somehow took the edge off the dizziness. I also thought these sessions shortened my recovery times after trips.

Sometime in July, the BPPN faded away—the crystals reabsorbed—and I was free of vertigo. Hallelujah! My mother came for a visit in early August, and I increased my activity to match my energy level. It felt wonderful to have some energy! There was a new performance art festival in Portland, in early September. Shelly and I attended four events, or at least the first half of four events. It was also the start of the symphony season and it was Rosh Hashanah. Even though I scaled back my participation to ninety minutes each of the two days, this was the beginning of the end of my "active" period.

October 3, 2003

I was laughing with Kay this morning about both of our tendencies to overdo—odd how it doesn't seem as funny when you're in the middle of the aftereffects. In the back of my mind I had a theory that by exposing myself to more frequent stimulus, perhaps I could still adapt. Even though I've accepted this illness, I still push at limits. When I was feeling poorly, I felt like a prisoner. It seemed I was constantly imprisoned by my physical limits. If I wanted to volunteer, what could I do? If I wanted to take a class? Join some group? But that's useless. It is what it is and there's no amount of frustration, anger or depression that will change it. All I can do is learn to thrive on what I can do—there is generally a way to find at least similar satisfaction and often deeper rewards. There is no use wishing this hadn't happened to me—I never do any more. I'm way past that. By now it's part of who I am.

With my usual determination I persevered and attended synagogue services during Yom Kippur. I wasn't depressed when I couldn't sleep for several days because of the dizziness and nausea. I decided to take the scientific approach and record each symptom in minute detail to determine how long it took me to recover. The most disturbing symptom was the jumpiness or vibration in my eyes whether they were open or closed. This jumpy vision made it hard to read or focus, and reading was one of my principal "down" time activities. After a week of dizziness with little or no head movement accompanied by noticeable ear and head pressure, I realized I was having a hydrops episode. Even the Zone Diet and my usual diuretic were unable to work their magic with the stress I had put my system under.

Several weeks later, as I was just starting to emerge from the hydrops episode, Shelly and I were first in line for flu shots. We were well aware that airplanes are famous germ incubators, and another trip to North Carolina was fast approaching. Right after the flu shot I started to feel even worse, and the vertigo from the BPPN started up again.

I saw Dr. Black and described the sequence of events. He immediately identified what happened. He reminded me that herpes was a constant factor in both the BPPN and hydrops episodes. I took daily Valtrex for the herpes, but this was no guarantee I would avoid an outbreak. In addition, the herpes could flare up without me knowing and still cause a hydrops or BPPN episode. Given this background, he thought the flu shot—or the flu shot and the ongoing hydrops—triggered a herpes flare-up that in turn triggered the BPPN.

The first and easiest step was to treat the BPPN. Colette came into the treatment room immediately and fitted me with the goggles to record the nystagmus, the eye movements. Then Dr. Black came and did the canalith repositioning procedure. I went home to be vertical for forty-eight hours. I also delayed the trip to North Carolina until December.

November 11, 2003

I've been feeling my limits, my losses, in a new, sadder way. The layers keep peeling away and I feel these demons again and again. I can see my acceptance of this illness—that it may get incrementally better or I may learn to manage it better but it's never going away—I can accept that and find some peace. On the other hand it doesn't mean a deep acceptance and peace permeate my life for all time. There are still struggles to understand who I am with these limits, why my life is meaningful. And yes, I know it is more meaningful now than before . . . I do.

The image that best calls forth how I feel is that I am blocked from joy—from loud, boisterous, irrepressible joy. I am blocked from moments of celebration, from moments of arms wide opened jubilation. My life is expressed in quiet small spaces, mostly alone. I yearn to laugh loudly, to have fun.

In the midst of feeling sorry for myself I had a long conversation with Gillie. It helped to say these things out loud. It helped tremendously to have vestibular friends to turn to. Gillie understood my frustrations but did not agree with my belief that everything happened in life for a reason. Her disagreement clarified my own strong beliefs.

I have always believed that the purpose of life, my life, was to learn and grow. Personal growth was one of my greatest joys. There was no denying that my balance problems were a clear gift in the personal growth arena. I was a more compassionate person, kinder and less focused on myself. The need to be praised, recognized, or more "successful" was a thing of my past. I had asked for growth and I was getting it from my life and yes, from my illness. If personal growth was my joy, then I was certainly not being "blocked from joy."

By late November the BPPN episode was over and I felt good again. Shelly and I made the planned trip to North Carolina to visit my mother and my sisters with no significant negative effects.

I headed into 2004 with optimism and a new resolve: to manage my limited energy more effectively, to use it in ways that were most rewarding to me. My hydrops and BPPN episodes in 2003 had been fewer and shorter than in previous years. I wanted to improve even more in 2004. I understood the cycles I kept repeating. I understood that if I wanted to feel "well" I needed to stay inside, largely alone, and do almost nothing. I understood that when I overdid it and experienced strong symptoms I wasn't simply ignoring my illness or failing to take a medication; I was making a choice to have a life, to do things that made life meaningful. I was aware that I hadn't found the balance yet, but I still believed it was possible.

Speaking From Experience: Tips to Make Your Journey Easier

1. The rapid, positive results I experienced from the Zone Diet in reducing my hydrops episodes were just short of miraculous. As a vegetarian for almost thirty years, I was convinced I was eating as healthy a diet as possible, so I was skeptical when I started on the Zone Diet. There are very few single actions that made as significant an impact on my life with vestibular disorders as changing to the Zone Diet. It is easy to check it out at www.zonediet.com. If you are interested in the science behind the diet, *The Zone* by Dr. Barry Sears is very helpful.

2. It was truly difficult to recognize hydrops episodes. First, the symptoms developed slowly; they tended to sneak up on me before I realized what was happening. Plus, one of the main symptoms—other than the obvious dizziness and general yucky nauseous feeling—was that the world got a bit foggy and confused; things got fuzzy. A further complication was that hydrops was unrelated to any specific motion or activity—like head position with BPPN or pressure with fistulas. Heat, dehydration, flu or cold, herpes—anything that raised my body temperature, whether I was aware of it or not—could cause a hydrops episode. Finally, hydrops episodes did not respond to treatment immediately; they resolved slowly, so it was never possible to say "Oh! I'm drinking more water and I feel better; it's hydrops." This confusion complicates life for patients with multiple vestibular problems.

3. I accepted that my vestibular disorders were a permanent part of my future. I no longer had illusions about one day getting well and forgetting I had ever struggled with vestibular disorders. However, I still wanted to improve my understanding of the disorders and to manage them to create as expansive a life as I could. In the midst of each struggle, each downturn, I couldn't help mourning the parts of life I missed and wished to experience again. It was in this light that I dreamed of moments of celebration and felt "blocked from joy." These feelings are a normal part of the transition to a different life. Acknowledge them and then turn your attention to the joys in your new life.

Suggested Reading

Sears, B. (1995). *The Zone: A Dietary Road Map to Lose Weight Permanently, Reset Your Genetic Code, Prevent Disease, and Achieve Maximum Physical Performance*. New York: HarperCollins.

20

A Giant Step Backward

The year 2004 started well on many fronts. I felt relatively symptom free and strong. I had both energy and motivation that had previously been in short supply. I wanted to build on the strength by doing further "energy work." There was a wealth of alternative healers and health practitioners in Portland, so I asked around for recommendations. Before too long the signs pointed to a neighbor who had moved to Portland several years earlier from a very successful practice in California. In late January I walked the few blocks to Gretchen's home for my first appointment, looking forward to a new experience that might possibly provide some further improvement, some greater stability in my health.

I explained my underlying balance problems as well as my hopes to find a treatment that would further enhance and strengthen my balance. The appointment was pleasant. It was subtle work largely involving laying hands on particular spots. Gretchen explained that she was working to balance the energy in my body at a deep level. I was enjoying the sensations and did not remember very much about the treatment except that when she started to work on my head she noticed a significant imbalance. She said I was likely to feel a bit spacey or tired for a few hours after the treatment, so I should take it easy. She was right. I was very dizzy and tired, but it cleared up overnight. The next appointment, a few weeks later, was going to involve a deeper treatment, and I looked forward to experiencing the positive effects; at the worst I assumed there would be no improvement.

One remark I made to Gretchen during the treatment caught her by surprise. I told her that I did not expect to "get well."

January 28, 2004

I felt she had some opinion or judgment about that remark or that attitude. And it's never bad to see that reflected and to check myself. I would love to be totally past this problem, to remove the limitations—and it isn't that I feel I don't have a right to hope. I've spent almost 8 years—8 years!—in this place and hoping was causing my life to feel second rate, not good enough, not authentic— as if I were waiting to get my real life back. Well, this is my real life. I accept it even while I make efforts to fine tune and improve. Acceptance isn't a closed thing, an end. It's a state of being and I like it here, it's more open to all possibilities.

In between appointments with Gretchen I decided to paint our attic bedroom—myself. The toughest part was painting the ceiling, I was very dizzy and unsteady looking up. There were also large pieces of furniture— dressers, the bed—that I needed to move ever so slightly to paint behind. I was careful about lifting because I was aware that strain put pressure on my ears that might reopen my fistulas. But honestly, how careful can you be lifting a dresser by yourself?

I went to my second appointment with Gretchen. As promised, she delivered a more intense treatment. For a grand finale she worked on my head for almost half an hour "rebalancing the energy in my brain," she said. I must admit I found this prospect frightening but I also believed her probability of success was very low. She made a few comments about how convoluted the current energy patterns were, and I wasn't sur- prised to hear it. After all, I had spent the last eight years spinning and whirling with various degrees of severity—that must have left some trace.

When I left Gretchen's house after this second appointment, I was severely dizzy—whirling. I wasn't overly concerned because it was the same pattern as before, and I assumed the dizziness would clear up by morning. It didn't. In fact, it was the start of ten days of severe dizziness, nausea, and blinding headaches. My sleep was disturbed again, and my usual medication was not helpful. Every time I was in a crowd or experienced motion I was agitated by a pulsing dizziness and constant strong movements inside my head.

In response, I dramatically curtailed my activity and started my recovery routines—a stricter Zone Diet, rest, meditate, sleep. I never went back to Gretchen. And I wondered again and again whether either the work with Gretchen or the moving of the dressers was the cause of my problems.

✳   ✳   ✳

Over the next few months I regularly felt okay when I was alone and resting but immediately felt terrible doing any activity involving crowds or motion. When I felt strong and optimistic, in January, I made a series of plans for trips and visits that I didn't want to cancel. They were the last shreds of a normal life, and I was determined to pursue them. First was a trip to Tucson, Arizona, a winter vacation with Shelly. Second, Jill and John's daughter Hannah was coming for a visit and bringing a friend. Both events were special experiences and well worth the aftereffects. I knew by now that my goal-oriented nature would carry me through the activity. I also knew I was going to crash afterward—and I did. This time, though, there was something different. The symptoms were definitely worse, and it took me longer to recover.

I also observed a new symptom—or, rather, I put a name to an old symptom. I described my recent experience to my vestibular friend, Kay: The world moved when I turned my head or moved my eyes when I had hydrops, but it also moved with my pulse, footfalls, swallowing, and heartbeat. Not dramatically, but subtly and noticeably. Kay confirmed that this was a pretty accurate description of what she called *oscillopsia*. No wonder she was nauseous and unable to walk very far if she had constant oscillopsia.

I kept waiting—wishing and hoping—for the symptoms to abate. I started the year feeling so healthy and strong, confident that the worst of my balance problems were behind me. Instead, I slipped slowly into the former flatness and exhaustion, worn out from the dizziness and nausea caused by trying to continue the pace of my life. It was time to admit I needed help.

I shared my observations with Dr. Black in late May. He agreed that the increased severity and persistence of symptoms required a thorough response. The best way to get a clear idea of what was going on this time was to repeat the balance testing. I did that over the next few weeks. During this May appointment I also sheepishly shared my experience with Gretchen and the energy balancing because I observed that the symptoms started dramatically after my second appointment. Both Dr. Black and Fran were more supportive of alternate techniques than I realized, but they urged me to work with professionals who were familiar with vestibular problems. Dr. Black reminded me that my brain and my balance system had accommodated and compensated for my balance problems, so "in balance" had a different meaning for me and for other vestibular patients. He didn't believe that my treatment from Gretchen was the cause of my current issues.

In early June, after I completed the balance tests, Shelly and I went together to hear the verdict. Dr. Black started by telling us that yet again, my hydrops was "out of control." The normal range for the indicator of excess fluid in the ear was 0.2, and my results were 0.72—a "very angry hydrops," in Dr. Black's terms. In fact, the hydrops was so severe Dr. Black suspected there was another, more serious underlying condition. The balance test results also indicated that both my eyes and my overall balance were affected by pressure and excess motion, which was unusual for a pure hydrops. The further possibilities included a reopened fistula in addition to a *dehiscence*—absence of bone—around my semicircular ear canal or an enlarged saccule, another part of the inner ear. My test results were not typical for a reopened fistula. The next step in diagnosis was to start ruling things out. A computerized tomography scan would rule out the dehiscence.

At the same time, Dr. Black prescribed a plan to control the hydrops that would also treat the potential for an enlarged saccule. He started me on a new diuretic, Hygroton, which he considered the best at controlling hydrops. He'd hesitated to prescribe Hygroton before because a very mild similar diuretic, spironolactone, had given me heart palpitations in 2000. (That's why I had been using a different drug, Diamox, for the last several years.) If I responded well to the Hygroton I was supposed to feel much better in three weeks. The other step in the plan was to explore more aggressive treatment of herpes. I was currently taking the daily recommended dose of Valtrex—the most aggressive treatment—and was unsure what else to do. My assignment was to contact my internist, my dermatologist, and my gynecologist to explore further options.

When Shelly and I returned in three weeks, the hydrops symptoms remained and the Hygroton was causing heart palpitations even though I took the potassium supplements as prescribed. After a blood test to confirm that my potassium levels were normal, Dr. Black increased the Hygroton dose and explained that with such severe hydrops it would take awhile longer for the small dose of diuretic to clear the excess fluid. At the same appointment he confirmed, on the basis of the computerized tomography scan, that there was no dehiscence, so we were dealing with either a reopened fistula, extreme hydrops, or an enlarged saccule.

We decided to focus on hydrops treatment as a next step. There are a range of treatments for hydrops, from conservative to destructive. The conservative treatments carry little or no associated risk and conserve the hair cells in the inner ear that are responsible for balance function. The destructive approaches are used only when there is no further hope of augmenting the function of the hair cells. Dr. Black had been trying to stick with conservative approaches. I had multiple conditions in each ear, which tends to reduce the effectiveness of many procedures. The following are my notes from this important session.

Diuretics: Along with the Zone Diet, diuretics are the first and most conservative step in hydrops treatment. Hygroton has been the most effective for vestibular conditions. I will start on a very low dose of Hygroton (25 mg every other day) and need to find the right balance with potassium. Dr. Black will check electrolytes continually and adjust the dosage of Hygroton and potassium. The usual next step would be 25 and 50 mg on alternating days. It could be another month before this dose level will impact the hydrops.

Perfusion: This procedure, done on an outpatient basis, works best for immune mediated hydrops and my hydrops appears to be viral mediated. The procedure involves cutting a small slit in the tympanic membrane and inserting a wick to deliver medication to the inner ear. Also, these steroid or anesthetic drops (perfusion) work best when only one ear is affected. Since there is little or no risk from the procedure it may be worth trying.

"Destructive" techniques: Streptomycin, gentamicin, and the other oto-toxic drug therapies are considered destructive techniques because they destroy the hair cells in the ears so that ear is not symptomatic. There is a fine line here in how far you can go in destroying hair cells before the process creates other symptoms that are worse than the present symptoms. Hearing loss is a significant risk. The standard is that this technique should not be undertaken unless the other ear is documented as normal.

Surgery: The specific surgical option—endolymphatic sac decompression—has a 70–80% chance of success and it needs to be repeated every two to fifteen years. This is not a high success rate, as most vestibular surgeries tend to exceed 95%. I am not a good candidate due to multiple symptoms in both ears.

Prosthetic device: Brain Port system. This is a new device that substitutes stimulation to the tongue for signals from the damaged parts of the vestibular system. It was developed last year at the University of Wisconsin and Dr. Black is doing a study to confirm the test results. However he is unsure of taking on more subjects at this point. When the device is commercially available patients would put it on every day or every few days for a short period of time and it removes many hydrops symptoms—dizziness, nausea, visual issues.

My friend Kay was currently undergoing treatment with streptomycin, a "destructive" technique. Her hydrops was severe, and her ears were detracting more than adding to her balance. It was an odd sort of all-or-nothing approach. If it worked, she would feel normal, like she felt before the balance problems. In the meantime she was in limbo, waiting and hoping that each streptomycin shot would be "the one." Her signal of success was that she would start to feel very dizzy and sick and then start to feel better. I used to end each conversation and each e-mail saying "Hope you feel truly terrible tomorrow." I did sincerely want her to get better; we were both rooting for each other.

Dr. Black's complete list of options was very helpful. Even in the midst of my hydrops fog I was comforted. We knew the alternatives and the risks associated with each step. The failure of a diuretic did not mean I would feel like this forever; there were more options to try. This was an important and timely understanding, because within a week the heart palpitations were severe and I went back to an elevated dose of my previous diuretic, Diamox. I also contacted my internist and went through a battery of heart tests, including an EKG, an echocardiogram, and a stress test. I even wore a halter monitor strapped around my chest for twenty-four hours to record real-time heart responses. I was thankful to learn that my heart was strong and healthy, just weirdly responsive to various diuretics.

Because I was touching all bases I also contacted Dr. Coffey, who had helped me with visual rehabilitation years before. He conducted a short form of the vision tests and identified one problem: gaze stabilization. This confirmed the findings of the balance tests as well. I was unable to hold a steady gaze, even with my head still, and when my head moved the world jumped wildly. Dr. Coffey shared his findings with Dr. Black as further information for diagnosis, but there was no rehabilitation available.

I made further progress with my dermatologist on the herpes front. She was at the forefront of treating herpes and recommended a higher dose, 1,000 mg daily, of Valtrex for unusually persistent herpes. She also recommended checking periodically to see if I continued to need such a high dose.

August 30, 2004

I'm pulling out all the stops, digging deep into my bag of tricks to get feeling better. Bringing on meditation and Morning Pages to add to my continuing better diet and renewed commitment to balance exercises. I've felt bad since February—not awful every day but never good and strong even for a whole day. I'm tormented by thoughts that the current diagnosis of hydrops isn't the whole picture—what if I reopened a fistula as well? What if it's another disease entirely? I'm also pressured by Shelly's (and yes, my) desire for a second expert opinion, a confirmation of the track we're on. It's a necessary step just to feel we've taken every avenue to understand this illness and reduce the symptoms. So in addition to feeling dizzy, nauseous, off balance and having headaches and joint aches—I am in an emotional turmoil. And yes, I'm depressed, more seriously than I have been in a few years. I got over it a month ago with a burst of anger but that outburst of rebellion only left me exhausted and more depleted. Like my dear friend Kay, I cannot imagine getting better any more.

Shelly and I spoke with Dr. Black about our thoughts on a second opinion, and he was very supportive and forthcoming with recommendations. For the time being, I was committed to the course we were on and wanted to pursue the two additional options: the Brain Port and the perfusion. My next step with Dr. Black was to try the Brain Port system or, as I called it "the tongue device." I was a questionable candidate, but Dr. Black allowed me in the research study because he wanted to provide me all the available conservative options.

While waiting for the Brain Port training Dr. Black recommended two additional tests: a platform pressure test and a tympanogram. The platform pressure test was the most definitive test, short of surgically opening the ear, for fistulas. During the test a tiny balloon was inflated in my outer ear as the balance platform moved underfoot. I tried to maintain balance with my eyes opened and then closed. The results of the pressure test were inconclusive but showed slightly stronger signs of a fistula.

The tympanogram, my first ever, was to measure the stiffness of the ear and to observe how much pressure applied during the platform test had an actual impact on my inner ear. The tympanogram showed that both my ears were relatively stiff, so the pressure was not being transferred to the inner ear. This made it more likely that my platform pressure test results indicated a reopened fistula.

September 17, 2004

Two recent tests are pointing to a reopened fistula, and at least that's a diagnosis, with a treatment. There is a surgery. But there are miles to go before I even think about that—"Brain Port" training that will take at least two weeks, and a consult about steroid perfusions versus fistula surgery. Meanwhile, I am nauseous, dizzy, have bad headaches, feel off balance, and am getting very sick in crowds. This is so pitiful it's laughable. I can't think of anything to do but stop talking about it and thinking about it—but I also know that is how I've lost focus on treatment in the past and let solutions slip away.

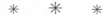

In the midst of these endless doctor's appointments and relentless symptoms, Shelly was in the final stages of selling his business, a process that had taken almost two years. The sale was extremely important to both of us. Even before I retired on disability we had always hoped to retire as early as possible and enjoy some very active years together. The sale was scheduled for early September, but last-minute issues caused a short delay and a big spike in Shelly's stress level.

We had anticipated this moment for years; it was the culmination of a decade of Shelly's professional life. In my imagination the sale was accompanied by a week-long celebration replete with parties and big announcements. The reality was quite different: last-minute hassles, keeping the sale confidential to make the announcement at the right moment, and concerns about how the employees would adapt. The sale started a countdown to his retirement; he'd agreed to work nearly full time as a consultant for a year and then part time for an additional year. He was too superstitious, too cautious, to celebrate early. His celebration took the form of slow exhalation, almost imperceptible mellowing and big doses of generosity to his employees and the new owners. The consummate professional, as always.

It was also the Jewish New Year, and my reflections focused on my continuing medical drama.

September 23, 2004

I need this year to be about completion on this balance front.
Pursuing all Dr. Black can offer aggressively and if I still feel a need,
seeking a second opinion. That's a large part of my focus for this
year—and the way I want that to be different is I want to learn and
grow in terms of inviting God, inviting my faith into that process.
I need so much help to lead me through with grace and clarity.
I want to be dedicated, purposeful, and positive. I want this to be a
learning experience—not just for me but for others around me. I can
live—and happily—with what I am able to do but I have to know
I tried—I didn't retreat.

Consistent with this auspicious time of breakthroughs—of endings and beginnings—Gillie was in the final stage of returning home to Israel. She continued to have serious balance problems, but we both understood that going home was more important than any vestibular treatment she could undertake. She needed to feel the support of her family and friends, to be able to work and to restart her life.

Dr. Black helped Gillie put together the travel arrangements because she could fly only on a medical flight. The damage to her ears was too severe to risk reopening her fistulas, and she needed to have the cabin pressurized to only 1,000 feet. The cabin pressure on a commercial flight is much higher—5,000 to 7,000 feet. The cost to get her to Israel was $100,000. Miraculously, her friends and family in Israel and Portland raised the necessary funds. She'd become quite a national cause in Israel. There were fundraising efforts on radio talk shows to help her get home, a unique version of one of the founding principles of the country—a place for Jews from around the world to come when they are in trouble.

Gillie courageously boarded the plane for the long flight in late September, entrusting her daughters to her sister and following Dr. Black's instructions to the letter. It was wonderful to hear her voice a few days after she arrived, sick but triumphant.

✳　　✳　　✳

In the spirit of trying all my options, I started the Brain Port training in mid-October. It was a unique and fascinating treatment. I wore a hat, more like a helmet, fitted with a gyroscope on top. The gyroscope sent signals about head tilt to a device I held in my mouth, on top of my tongue.

The device was teaching my tongue to assume the balance functions my ears were not performing. For this training I stood, eyes closed, on a six- inch-thick piece of foam. Under ordinary conditions I couldn't stand, even with my eyes open, on a six-inch block of foam, so this alone was impressive.

The benefits of the Brain Port were apparent within one to two sessions for patients with no balance function. The results were less clear for patients like me whose balance functions were impaired by hydrops or fistulas. I enjoyed the sessions; they were powerful standing meditations, and I experienced short-term energy boosts afterward. Over the week, though, I became more and more fatigued, and my basic symptoms were unchanged. Dr. Black stopped the test. I was not disappointed or let down, but I did begin to get myself emotionally ready for another six to twelve months of down time to treat the suspected fistula.

The next step in our grand plan was the perfusion. The first stop was to see Dr. Epley for a labyrinthine anesthesia test (LAT). Dr. Epley routinely performed these LATs and subsequent perfusions. The LAT was truly fascinating. Dr. Epley made a small incision in my right ear and placed medication—both steroid and anesthetic—into my middle ear. I was to observe symptoms carefully, particularly noting the time symptoms started and stopped. If I felt better quickly but the effects wore off in twelve to forty-eight hours, it was most likely due to the anesthetic. If the positive effects were longer lasting, it was most likely the steroid. Either way, we'd have a treatment!

The LAT was done late in the day, and I thought I felt better before I went to sleep, but I was unsure. I woke up the next morning feeling happy, chatty, energetic, and animated, and moving my head. I actually started to cry, I felt so good. It was such a sharp contrast to how I usually felt, how I'd felt only twelve hours before. It was like stepping into an alternate reality.

My tears were from sorrow and joy: sorrow for the loss of this energetic, animated person who'd disappeared eight years ago, and joy from the momentary wonder of feeling great and the possibility of feeling this way again in the future. The next step was to insert a micro-wick and start a perfusion, a dripping, of the anesthetic into my ear. I could not wait! The possibility of feeling like this every day was beyond my wildest dreams.

Three hours later I started to feel very, very bad—too dizzy to walk. I felt so bad I had to delay my appointment with Dr. Epley to insert the wick and start treatment. While I was recovering from the LAT I was instructed to put in earplugs while showering. After two days I noticed that when I inserted the plug—and when I pulled it out—I was spinning and tilting wildly. Something clicked. This was strong evidence of symptoms with pressure; this was a fistula!

I e-mailed Dr. Black, and he called me within ten minutes. He stopped the planned perfusion because he was certain I had an opened fistula. Any additional steroid would compromise healing of the wound if I decided to proceed with surgery. It wasn't until after we talked that I remembered Dr. Black told me that the LAT would cause severe symptoms if I had an opened fistula. The anesthetic and steroid would go through my middle ear into my inner ear. Confirmations of the fistula diagnosis were coming in fast and furious. Without a great deal of additional deliberation, Shelly and I decided surgery was the right next step, and we scheduled it for December 15.

Over the next few weeks Shelly and I took trips to Los Angeles and to North Carolina. These were the last trips I would be able to take for a year because it took that long for the fistula to heal sufficiently to withstand the pressure of flying I began to have some doubts about the surgery or, more accurately, some dread. It was easy to lose track of how bad I now felt and start to question the need for surgery. Like so many times before, I'd been dizzy and nauseous for so long it began to feel normal. It was also hard to dissociate bed rest from the bed rest I'd endured after Dad's death seven years earlier.

December 14, 2004

*Of course I hope the surgery goes well and the fistula closes. I hope
I am successful in healing the wound and getting new stronger ears.
I also hope I can feel as well as I felt a year ago before the setback. It
is beyond my imagination that I also might go to synagogue and be
in a crowd again—and I understand that travel will always be a risk.
But these are my hopes—no matter how hard I push them into the
background. And no matter how depressed or sad, my intention is to
do all I can to be better—and to do it with all my heart and dedication.*

When we returned home after the trips I made final preparations for the bed rest after surgery—dog walkers, help with grocery shopping and cooking, help with laundry. There were also the hospital preparations and interviews that made the upcoming surgery more and more real. Before I knew it December 15 had arrived and I was prepped and ready.

Dr. Black explained that I would be under anesthesia but he needed me to be awake and alert. After being wheeled into the surgical room, the next thing I knew I was in recovery. The anesthesiologist checked on me and asked how I was doing. He chuckled when he told me I had talked up a blue streak in the operating room, asking Dr. Black essentially the same question every few minutes: "Did you find anything? What do you see in there?"

When Dr. Black came to my hospital room a few hours later he was beaming from ear to ear. After years of speculation, he'd seen the fistula and he now understood all the variable test results and uncertain diagnoses. I had a rare, congenital condition called *Okano's microfissure*, which involves a vestigial opening that used to contain a blood vessel. This opening runs through and weakens the *round window*, one of two membrane-sealed openings in the inner ear. (The other is called the *oval window*.) These are where fistulas occur. This weakening made the ear very susceptible to a tear, a fistula.

> Okano's microfissure is a rare, congenital condition that involves a vestigial opening that used to contain a blood vessel. The opening runs through and weakens the round window, one of two membrane-sealed openings in the inner ear. (The other is called the oval window.) These are where fistulas occur.

Dr. Black confirmed that I didn't stand a chance of getting better without surgery. The fistula had probably opened and closed frequently over the years. During surgery, he plugged the opening and patched both the oval and round windows. With the patches, my right ear was stronger than it had ever been in my life. I barely registered when he mentioned it was likely I had a similar condition in my left ear. I refused to worry about anything new.

Speaking From Experience: Tips to Make Your Journey Easier

1. It was really disappointing to have a serious setback—to feel worse after eight years of treatment. However, my experience in identifying and tracking symptoms was a huge advantage. Specifically, my symptom tracking after the brain port sessions expedited the conclusion that it was not working and resulted in an end to the treatment. My reporting of symptoms after the LAT confirmed the fistula and prevented risks from steroid perfusion. These were concrete rewards. At some point you will become "professional" patient—you will know the healing routines and will be managing your vestibular disorders. There will probably still be setbacks, but you will be able to address them and weather them more effectively.

2. Similarly, my role as manager of my medical team matured and paid dividends. Interactions with Dr. Black were pragmatic and analytic. In each session there was a list of tests he needed me to take for his review. In addition, there were contacts I needed to make with other doctors to coordinate my care with my vestibular issues. We were following a plan of moving from least to greatest risk treatment to identify and address the fundamental problem.

21

Finding Balance

DECEMBER 2004–OCTOBER 2006

This bed rest was both physically and emotionally different, and I knew it immediately. Emotionally, I was at peace with both my father's death and the end of my career. No other huge emotional issues loomed to weigh me down. Physically, it made a world of difference to have the surgery both confirm and repair the fistula. This certainty that the fistula was closed and the knowledge that the bed rest was essential to heal the surgical patch was a major sea change. It was also much less frightening because of my knowledge about vestibular problems—with eight years under my belt, I felt like a professional.

Of course, there were the usual ups and downs. For the first month or so I had a serious hydrops episode that caused constant, severe dizziness. Dr. Black's nurse, Fran, called regularly and assured me that this hydrops was normal. Postclosure hydrops was a positive indicator that the surgical patch was holding. The patch dammed the excess fluid building up, and this condition would resolve in time if I stayed on the Zone Diet, took my diuretic, and drank water regularly. These periodically recurring hydrops episodes confused the healing process because it still took me awhile to realize that the symptoms were hydrops related.

For the first few weeks I watched my hearing closely. There were loud whooshing sounds in my right ear almost constantly. I was told these would decrease significantly and might even go away entirely. The real concern was a sudden drop or change in hearing. Hearing loss was one of the highest risks of surgery, but if we caught it early enough there were remedies Dr. Black could try.

For the first six weeks I was both allowed and encouraged to be up and around for ninety minutes a day. Included in this total were my daily shower and the extreme challenge of getting down two flights of stairs and back up again, a task I only attempted after a week at home. The major focus of bed rest was to avoid putting any pressure on my ear that could weaken or tear the surgical patch. I slept on a wedge, practically sitting up. I got my share of headaches, which my chiropractor friend Paul was able to treat. The most alarming event of the first six weeks was my inadvertent sneeze—forbidden on bed rest because of the sudden pressure on the patch. I freaked out about this for a few hours but was reassured after I called Fran. Every time I overdid things and got symptoms I sat myself back down and regrouped.

Despite the enforced solitude and the erratic hydrops episodes, I was healing faster than my previous bed rest experience. By the second stage of bed rest—weeks six through twelve—I felt stronger, and my symptoms were less intense. Fortunately, I had detailed notes tracking symptoms from the previous bed rest for comparison. I still experienced symptoms with each new activity, but I bounced back quickly and made steady progress. My appointment with Dr. Black to check in on my progress confirmed my observations. He supported my increased activity level as long as I stopped and rested when any symptoms arose.

It helped to go back and read my notes about the first bed rest, so I easily remembered that the further I moved from complete inactivity the more challenging it was. Whether it was walking or driving, each new activity was accompanied by the expectation of an immediate return to normalcy. The better I felt, the better I wanted to feel. This was my old friend, goal-oriented Sue, pushing for the finish line.

The only major setback in my recovery from surgery occurred in mid-March at my check-in with Dr. Black after the second six weeks. I'd tried to sleep on two pillows rather than the huge wedge (well, it seemed huge to me). Every time I tried to sleep without the wedge I woke up very nauseous with a very bad headache. Dr. Black immediately said it sounded like there was a leak in the left ear. Because I'd had surgery on the right ear, a left ear leak was very bad news. This wasn't the first time I reported a symptom that hinted at a left ear fistula, but this was the most certainty I had heard from Dr. Black. Although there were far more encouraging reports in the six week review, this one comment haunted me.

Over the next few weeks I stuck closely to my routines. I meditated on some sage advice I cherished, and tried to follow, from my father, "If you can do something about it, do it! Don't sit around and worry about it." So I prayed. And then Shelly and I reviewed all our notes and decided, based on our own knowledge and observations, my symptoms indicated a benign paroxysmal positional nystagmus episode that we couldn't verify yet. In this stage of bed rest I couldn't lie flat to check for spinning. This was the best we could do for now.

My progress slowed, as it typically did, in stage three of the bed rest. At the same time I was beset with some normal medical problems, including a bladder infection. With these challenges on top of the fear about a left ear fistula, I allowed myself to think deeply about what my future might hold.

March 31, 2005

The whole thing about expectation is so seductive. No matter how low I set my expectations I still manage to be disappointed. It seems to be impossible to try any treatment with detachment—truly not expecting a positive result but being open to it. Being "open to" is clearly the crack that hope sneaks through. But without being open to it, I probably wouldn't try at all. So many paradoxes. I accept on a deep level that I have these balance problems—that they will always be a part of my life. I do not expect to look back at some point in the future and say . . . "Oh, I forgot about that, that was a rough period." . . . This does not feel like a phase that will end. I accept that. At the same time it feels reasonable to try to feel better if at all possible. The trap is that the trying consumes your life, alters it, becomes it. I can more readily understand those people who just disappear, stay inside and feel better, live within their limits. I never understood them before but I do now. It's not my make-up, I believe in solutions, I would always wonder if I were overlooking an answer. But at some point the game has to be over, maybe that is what has been eating at me—the game seems to stretch endlessly before me again—if I don't start to feel better it's probably the left ear, or there is always the anesthesia test and steroid treatment . . . or, or, or.

As I was walking today I had another thought I've had a hundred times—Why can't I just push through it? What's so tough about being dizzy and nauseous? Why cower so from those symptoms? Why not just push through and do whatever it is I want to do and ignore the symptoms? I try that approach from time to time—in moments of rebellion and self-destruction—and for a little while it feels good, free. Ultimately systems "shut down" but it's good for awhile.

I chose this surgery and this long recovery and it's not as difficult as before. This time is less confusing. These feelings and cycles are purer—and it's still hard. So why is that? Why do I say it's hard? Aside from feeling physically bad—depressed, nauseous, tired, with this damnable ringing in my ears all the time, I feel pitiful and pitiable—the shut in, the sick person. I'm not good at being needy. It's psychically and emotionally difficult to feel so limited, so inactive, so uncertain. I've always had a self-concept as someone who is active, powerful, purposeful, a seeker and searcher for meaning—determined, decisive, independent. Just listing these things makes it clear why this is hard—it challenges everything I believe about myself.

Well, not everything. There is a part of me that knows I can have a meaningful life, still make a contribution and enrich the lives of others, even if I never leave the house. I can have a rich interior life. In fact I value the silence and solitude and the depth of peace I find here. At the core again is balance, balance in all aspects. I want (I need?) to be able to go out, to be active, to have experience—and I want to be able to pause, reflect and integrate that experience. I want an external life and an internal life. I want to keep living and growing based on new ideas and inputs. Yes, I can do that from inside the house—but do I have to? I guess that is the question.

As so often happened, the physical downturn and the deep reflections were followed by a steady and sustained uphill climb. Many years before, Dr. Lin had spent hours during our acupuncture sessions educating me about the cyclical nature of the healing process. It is not a straight line. It's more like a spiral staircase. Often the moments that appear to be valleys or setbacks are when energy is being gathered for the next climb. These reflections gave me a different perspective and a foundation on which to build. I moved cautiously through each stage of the bed rest, trying new activities and stopping when I had symptoms, then trying again. At close range, this felt like ups and downs, but with a little perspective I could see there was steady progress over the weeks and months. I gained confidence that the surgery was a success, and there were no further signs of an immediate problem with my left ear.

> The healing process is cyclical in nature. It is not a straight line. It's more like a spiral staircase. Often the moments that appear to be valleys or setbacks are when energy is being gathered for the next climb.

My progress was so rapid Shelly and I were able to start our trips to Bend in July: over the mountains only seven months after surgery! That was the good news; the bad news was the travel symptoms were reduced from last year with the opened fistula but still definitely a limiting factor. Still, simply sitting by the river under the bright blue sky, being in this serene place, was a substantial reward. I felt wonderful and strong when we were hiking around the mountain lakes; this was so different from dragging myself through life. The trip back was harder. Coming down from a higher altitude meant moving into greater barometric pressure and that exacerbated my travel-related dizziness and nausea and the delayed-motion sensation. I recovered in a week, but the symptoms got my attention and I resolved to find some way to make progress on the *mal de debarquement*.

During the next several months I resumed a more and more normal life and noted my symptoms in detail. Crowds were definitely still a problem, especially when combined with noise. Even if I wore ear plugs throughout the event it was no help. My only strategy was avoidance. I experienced severe hydrops symptoms in the fall. Dr. Black gently reminded me how recently, in vestibular terms, I'd had surgery. I was still susceptible to a post-closure hydrops. There was no need for concern; it should resolve on its own, about a year to a year and a half after surgery. That would be June 2006!

In the same week I was talking with another vestibular friend and she told me, for the first time, that she had been through five fistula surgeries. She told me she continued to improve for eighteen months after each surgery. My first reaction to June 2006 had been impatience, incredulity at having to wait so long. Now I saw that I could continue to feel better and better over the next nine months and that was all good. It was so very helpful to have these benchmarks, from Dr. Black and confirmed by a fellow patient.

*   *   *

I was living a full life again, filled with travel, social engagements, and the normal daily tasks. I was painting, gardening, and walking regularly. With the fistula closed, there were days it was possible to feel good. When I overdid activity, especially in the heat or during barometric swings, I felt bad again. The fistula symptoms were far more dramatic and there was a sense of deadness, lifelessness, and lack of motivation that came with the fistula. Those dramatic symptoms were gone and the more familiar transitory dizziness, nausea, and headaches resumed. As I recorded my symptoms, again, I wished for more words to describe dizziness and nausea. As I knew them they were multidimensional, many faceted.

I was compiling a medical chronology—a listing of all my medical appointments with an explanation of symptoms, diagnoses, and treatment. I unearthed a series of suggestions Dr. Black had made over the years, eight years and counting. I realized there were quite a few helpful ideas I hadn't heard, or hadn't responded to, the first time. I was also struck by the patterns of my symptoms, the repetition of episodes and the predictability of severe symptoms.

As a direct result of preparing this chronology I began to develop a method for charting activity and assigning points to each activity. Shelly was instrumental in pointing out that my symptoms were clearly worse when I was too active and that the type of activity influenced the severity of the symptoms. For years, I had listed my daily symptoms as a way to avoid losing track of how I felt. I had never before tracked my activity levels and tried to correlate activity and symptoms.

I started by listing the activities I knew were challenging: shopping, movies, using the computer for more than an hour, eating out, driving or riding in a car for more than an hour, synagogue services, airplane flights, and entertainment. I knew if I kept my involvement under an hour for most of these activities, the symptoms would be less. I would recover more rapidly. I developed a point system that reflected higher points for a longer exposure. For example, a flight to Los Angeles was two hours, so I assigned it four points. The flight to North Carolina was eight hours, so I assigned ten points. At first I guessed about the points, but as I made these guesses I realized I understood the impact of activities quite well. I'd simply never bothered to quantify it.

Over the next weeks and months, I recorded my activity points every day. At the bottom of the chart I also summarized my overall nausea and dizziness level. If I recorded low-level dizziness or nausea—one or two on a scale of one to ten—that day was a good one and received an "A" overall. My worst symptom days were recorded as "D"s. On those days, all my symptoms were worse than six on a scale of one to ten. Very soon I was able to see that charting activities, and keeping track of my energy expenditures, was a valuable management tool. If I pulled out the chart and saw a week full of Ds on the symptom summary line, it was clear I should keep my activity to a minimum, fewer than five or six points, over the next few days.

It wasn't a surprise to see that when I overextended myself I felt bad. What was a surprise was that the ability to see the results laid out for each month made an important impact on my life. The daily discipline of recording symptoms and activities and then examining them side by side provided the perspective I needed to take greater control of my life. I looked at the chart every day and was reminded of the need to manage my activity every day. As a result, I felt less like I was a victim of my limits and much more in control of how I decided to use my energy and manage my symptoms. I was more actively engaged in tailoring a solution for myself.

February 21, 2006

I am grateful for the peace and fullness flowing back. I see how I was/am forcing a faster rhythm on my life—super-imposing a faster pulse and a shallower breath. I need slow and deep at least for a while. Today while I was meditating I caught a glimpse of my "path." Not surprisingly, it was an animal path or a disused footpath. I say not surprising because the main roads are behind me now— school, career—like others who are retiring my oath is uncharted, individual. This image helped me to see why I pause and feel like I'm wandering around at times. The path is faint and sometimes I find I am following a streambed not a path. At those times I need to pause and collect myself to reach some clarity. Charging through unmarked terrain, bushwhacking, is an illusory path. I believe there is a path I should follow, I am still a seeker after all.

Beginning to see myself as a retiree as opposed to a sick person also was a major step.

Over the next six months, I went to Dr. Black several times. First, Shelly and I wanted to share our progress with tracking activities and symptoms. As a result of the tracking we had identified the need for options to address crowd-related motion and travel motion. We were well aware that I'd already tried every possible medication for my motion sickness in crowds. We were also aware that there was no known treatment for *mal de debarquement* except not doing whatever brought it on. Finally, we knew Dr. Black was often able to pull a rabbit out of his hat—when you least expected it, he would provide a new insight of great value.

Dr. Black was intrigued by the new activity and symptom tracking. It did not meet the standard for scientific data, but he described several research attempts to better define and quantify symptoms like dizziness and nausea. The real surprise was his next suggestion. One of his colleagues at NASA (the space flight guys) had developed goggles to address motion sickness in crowds. Dr. Black was an advisor to NASA and was on NASA's balance research team. He regularly used what he learned from that in his practice. He actually had a pair of goggles in the office. He wanted me to test them for a few weeks and note each situation, as well as my symptoms, while I had the goggles on. The term *goggles* was slightly off-putting, I wasn't enthusiastic about looking like a Star Wars character. Regardless, I was excited to give the goggles a try.

It turned out that *goggles* was a slight misnomer. *Strobe sunglasses* was a more descriptive term. The glasses were big and black, like lab glasses. There was a nickel-sized battery on one side, and when it was inserted the glasses flashed wildly on the inside part that faced my eyes.

April 25, 2006

Here are some headlines from the past few weeks. First, Dr. Black and his strobe glasses have to be recorded as a triumph. I have a new sense of confidence about going into a crowd with the glasses. Yes, the strobe is disturbing but the disturbance is worth it. I have no motion sickness in crowds for an hour or an hour and a half. I've worn the glasses to Passover dinners, restaurants, movies, a dance performance and shopping. They are effective. The darkness and flashing limit my abilities at some venues (grocery shopping, ordering in a restaurant) but generally this is a major development.

When friends saw the strobe lights flashing in my glasses they always asked if there were any side effects from wearing them. Shelly liked to tease them (and me!) that "other than the Tourette-like side effect of Sue periodically jumping up without warning and starting to disco dance, it was all good." In the spring when we went to a baseball game, I noticed a young guy looking in my direction. He got up and walked over to tell me "Your glasses rock!!!" Apparently they're hip-looking to a certain audience.

During this same period I worked on my *mal de debarquement* as well, developing a better description of symptoms, charting the frequency and severity of, and experimenting with techniques to relieve symptoms. Trips to Bend were a predictable source of symptoms to ponder and list. I always had a sensation I was still moving after the trip, but this movement was a minor part of the overall syndrome. These posttrip symptoms lasted five to seven days.

February 28, 2006

I feel indescribably awful after the drive. Not that it is so painful or so physically trying—there are literally no words in my vocabulary to describe it. I feel apart from myself, disengaged, like a zombie—skin crawling, I just want whatever it is to stop. "It" makes me feel off balance and like I don't want to move my head at all. Like there is an absence of my normal internal rhythm moving my limbs in a coordinated way. And I feel locked up—no words come to mind, I can't focus, can't really speak. Just the barest essentials take all my energy. The dizziness is a sign I am beginning a return, a recovery.

Shelly and I experimented with walking midway through a trip, after an hour and a half of the drive. There were many wilderness parks and hiking trails along the route, and we planned two-mile hikes to break up the drive. Bunkee was thrilled with this new approach, but I didn't notice any difference in my symptoms. During this same period, I also experimented with chiropractic adjustments and cranial work. After each drive back to Portland, I went to Paul for an immediate adjustment. We found that these adjustments were a good start but did not clear up my physical problems. Paul suggested I come back the next day for a further adjustment and some cranial work to complete the rebalancing. This two-day treatment approach made a significant impact: It cut my recovery time in half.

By September, I was ready to approach Dr. Black with my findings, organized in matrix form listing every trip to Bend. I tracked fifteen symptoms after each drive and identified the most frequent and severe: dizziness/vertigo, off balance/legs disconnected from body, nausea, vibration/motion, locked up/flat/can't talk, headache, insomnia, and fatigue. I also recorded the recovery time for each trip; it was generally five to seven days, or two to four days with chiropractic adjustment.

When we saw Dr. Black in September 2006, he was immediately intrigued. These data were much richer and led him to more specific responses than my past general complaints about *mal de debarquement*. Dr. Black said *mal de debarquement* was poorly understood, and he detailed for me and Shelly his concept of the physical mechanisms at work. He used the word *entrain* to describe how my body took on the motion of the vehicle or the airplane and continued to experience that motion even after it had stopped. He suggested that the best approach to minimize the symptoms was to disrupt entrainment—to break the force and influence of the motion. Shelly described our inability to find any positive impact from the mid-trip walks. Dr. Black thought the walks were too much like the rhythm of the car and suggested throwing a ball or doing calisthenics. He was also very interested in the benefits I observed from chiropractic adjustments and cranial work.

This conversation was the origin of a self-designed remedy I called the "witch doctor dance," my personal version of vestibular disco. After every hour of driving, we stopped and I got out of the car and did a set of strange gyrations for two minutes. The gyrations started as jumping jacks and mutated into a wild throwing about of arms and legs while running in place or jumping up and down. Oddly enough, it helped. Within a few trips of perfecting the technique, my symptoms were less severe and, perhaps more important, I recovered in two to three days rather than five to seven. When combined with the chiropractic treatments, I was often able to recover in one to two days. If someone posts a video of a crazy woman dancing on the Mount Hood pass, you'll know it's me.

The witch doctor dance was a difficult maneuver in an airplane lavatory, but I can tell you that it IS possible. The dance was not quite as effective in the plane, probably because the motion and noise of the plane are more forceful, easier to entrain, and I couldn't escape it, even when I was dancing—I couldn't exactly leave the plane midflight. However, the general effect was the same: My symptoms were less severe and they cleared up more rapidly.

There was one lingering issue: the recurring episodes of benign paroxysmal positional nystagmus (BPPN) and associated vertigo were hanging on longer and longer. Although there were things that could be done to address BPPN, the actions often failed to work for me. On a recent visit, Dr. Black pulled another rabbit from his hat and offered a clue: There was some early scientific speculation about a BPPN link to osteopenia and calcium mobilization. It might or might not pan out, but I was sure of one thing: I was intrigued. With the lighthearted spirit of a junior gumshoe, I made the call to the leading osteoporosis specialist in Portland. I don't know where this next clue will lead; time will tell.

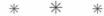

It was impossible to ignore this trifecta of positive developments: charting the activity and symptoms, the strobe glasses, and the witch doctor dance. Nothing was a silver bullet. It was a weird combination of odds and ends that strangely enough made a difference. I pulled out my chart of vestibular problems and associated remedies to update it and realized I now had a management strategy for every one of my problems—fistulas, hydrops, BPPN, crowd motion, travel motion, insomnia, and *mal de debarquement*. These were not cures, but they provided me some ability to manage my way through the symptoms. Most of the actions were preventative, such as restrictions on lifting for fistulas, or the Zone Diet and diuretic for hydrops, or Valtrex for herpes prevention. Other actions involved medications that lessened the severity of symptoms, like Phenergan for travel and insomnia. And then there were the new actions: the glasses, the witch doctor dance, and the activity/symptom charting.

I was not kidding myself. My balance disorder was not fixed; I was not well in the traditional sense. However, as I reflected on the concept of being well, I realized I was better than well. I was transformed.

October 10, 2006

I've had two interesting reflections—first about acceptance. Although I know in my heart and soul what that means, I'm hard pressed to express the concept in words. It certainly is not surrender or giving up—because it has no negative or diminishing connotation. More like a friendship or a family—where you know someone so very well you can predict their behavior—the good and the disappointing—and you see it all as a part of the whole that you love. Without this illness, which can definitely try your soul, I would not have many riches in my life—slow pace, deep relationships, introspection, growing patience, vulnerability. I am interested in learning more about the concept of acceptance. Perhaps that learning will enhance the depth of my appreciation and understanding of my own acceptance. It seems like an open door I want to walk through.

Secondly, Shelly and I saw Dr. Black today . . . As we drove home, I realized I no longer feel like a helpless patient—a victim of the illness. I feel more like a partner in research with Dr. Black. Part of this is my own growth and acceptance and part of it is Dr. Black. He has been such a wonderful doctor—I am so grateful for his knowledge and his caring nature. This door also seems open—filled with meaningful possibilities—ways I might help others with this illness through my connection with Dr. Black.

If one of life's major challenges is to know ourselves, then there is a rich source of self-knowledge through illness and healing. My own healing slowed me down so I could see things I would have missed at my previous pace. I experienced healing as miraculous. That we are given the gift of physical bodies with the capacity to heal, that we have the gift of intelligence to understand the working of our bodies, that we have the benefit of others who dedicate themselves to healing—all these things were wondrous.

Whatever the future holds, I am grateful for the journey.

Speaking From Experience: Tips to Make Your Journey Easier

1. The last two additions to my vestibular tool kit—activity and symptom tracking and the witch doctor dance—were personal inventions. These inventions were the fruits of years of hard work at studying and finally understanding my symptoms. It is not possible to say for sure that these tools will work for every vestibular patient. However, I know all patients can advance their progress by taking an active role in their care, experimenting with activities and solutions, and closely monitoring their symptoms.

2. I must offer a word about time in regard to vestibular disorders. When you think about how complex the vestibular systems is—brain, eyes, ears, muscles, and joints—it is understandable that small problems can be magnified and that corrections need time to work through the system. I developed a rule of thumb about vestibular healing: No matter how much patience I called on in setting up reasonable timelines, the time to heal always exceeded my patience. This is actually good news. The healing proceeds slowly, and the full results of treatment may not be apparent for a long time—years, even.

3. Entering the world of the chronically ill was like moving to a foreign country: I needed to learn the language, familiarize myself with new customs, develop new friendships, and adapt my life to a totally strange situation. The best advice I can offer to anyone with vestibular problems is this: Don't give up. Keep trying to find a path that works for you, a path that can turn this foreign country into your new home.

Epilogue

by Dr. F. Owen Black

There are some important resources available to patients with vestibular disorders. The Internet can connect patients with many websites.

- The National Institutes of Health provides the most reliable research references: http://www.ncbi.nlm.nih.gov/sites/entrez. This website is considered to be one of the most scientifically reliable because most of the information has been peer reviewed.
- The Vestibular Disorders Association of America (VEDA): http://www.vestibular.org. This website provides patient-focused information.

A word of caution is in order when using information from the numerous websites available. Always review any information obtained from a website with your licensed health care professional before implementing any recommendations obtained from a website.

Suggested Reading:

1. Eggers SDZ & Zee DS. Vertigo and Imbalance: Clinical Neurophysiology of the Vestibular System. In Daube JR & Mauguière F, Eds. *Handbook of Clinical Neurophysiology*. Boston: Elsevier, 2010.

   Comment: This text reviews the most common vestibular disorders and their treatment.

2. Hanes DA & McCollum G. Cognitive-vestibular interactions: A review of patient difficulties and possible mechanisms. *Journal of Vestibular Research 16* (2006) 75–91. Amsterdam: IOS Press.

   <u>Comment</u>: Ms. Hickey's description of her cognitive problems is not unique amongst patients with vestibular disorders. This paper reviews some current concepts regarding disruption of cognition associated with vestibular disorders.

Index